# Prescription
# for Bankruptcy

*A doctor's perspective on America's failing
health care system and how we can fix it*

**Edward P Hoffer, MD
FACP, FACC, FACMI**

OMNI PUBLISHING CO.
2018

Published by
Omni Publishing Co.
www.omni-pub.com
September 2018


**Library of Congress cataloging-in-publication data**
Hoffer, Edward P.
Prescription for Bankruptcy: A doctor's perspective on America's
failing health care system and how we can fix it

ISBN: 978-0692171486

This book is dedicated to the memory of my parents,
Wynne and Arthur Hoffer, who were always loving and
supportive and who fostered a life-long love of learning.

# Table of Contents

# Introduction

The US health care system is badly broken.

We spend much more per capita on health care than any other country on earth and yet our national health statistics are nowhere near the top. We spend twice the average of comparable countries, yet by many measures—percentage of uninsured, life expectancy, maternal and infant mortality—we lag well behind.

In 2017, the US population was 324 million and the Centers for Medicare and Medicaid Services (CMS) estimated that our national health spending had reached $3.5 trillion, for a per capita spending of $10,800. Our national health spending was 31 percent higher than in Switzerland, our closest "competitor." Per capita spending on health care by comparable developed countries is generally half that of the US: Germany $5,550, Netherlands $5,385, Belgium $4,800, Canada $4,750, France $4,600. As a percentage of the nation's gross national product we are equally bad. In the US it is nearly 18 percent, while in the comparable developed countries it is a bit over 10 percent. At the current rate of health care inflation, health care spending is projected to represent 19.9 percent of gross domestic product by 2025.

Perhaps a difference of 8 percent does not sound overwhelming, so let me put that in perspective. The United States GDP last year was almost $20 trillion. If we were to cut the health care system's 18 percent down to the 10 percent that is the average of other Western democracies, we would save $1.6 trillion annually. In three years, we would save enough money to repair—entirely—America's failing infrastructure. Every day in the United States, there are on average 657 water main breaks and our bridges are collapsing. We could rebuild all our highways, roads and bridges; rebuild our electrical grid; repair our schools, dams and ports. That is what 8 percent could do!

This wildly excessive spending **might** be acceptable if we were proportionally healthier, but we are far from it.

A baby born in the United States in 2016 had a life expectancy of 78.6 years. Newborns in 29 other countries in that year had a life expectancy of more than 80 years. In Japan, life expectancy at birth was 83.7; in Singapore and Switzerland 83.4; Austria 82.8; Spain 82.6.

The US has poorer child health outcomes than other wealthy nations. In a 2013 article on the US health care system, *Time Magazine* reported that a child born in Havana, Cuba, had a better chance of living to age two than a child born in the United States! A study published in *Health Affairs* in January 2018 found that among 20 OECD nations, the risk of death in the US was greater than the average—76 percent greater for infants and 57 percent greater for children aged one to 19—even though we have many more neonatal intensive care units per capita than these other countries. (The OECD, or Organization for Economic Co-operation and Development, is an intergovernmental economic organization with 35 member-countries, founded in 1961 to stimulate economic progress and world trade. Its member countries are primarily "western democracies," and include the United States, Canada, Australia, Japan, South Korea and most European countries. The OECD is often used as a comparison source when studying health care, as none of its members has the economic development issues that would make health care less important than basic needs such as food and housing.)

A report published by the Commonwealth Fund in 2017 compared the performance of the health care systems in 11 rich democracies ranging from Australia to the United States. The US ranked dead last. Only in the category of care process was the US in the middle (fifth). It ranked last in access, equity and health care outcomes, and tenth in administrative efficiency.

As documented in a *USA Today* report in July 2018, the maternal death rate in the United States is dramatically worse than it is in other developed nations. In 2015, the maternal death rate per 100,000 live births was 6.4 in Japan; 7.3 in Canada; 7.8 in France; 8.8 in the United Kingdom; 9 in Germany; and a staggering 26.4 in the US. Moreover, the rate has been falling in all of these countries except the US, where it has increased significantly.

Unlike in most developed countries, where adequate health care for all is routinely available and rarely causes financial hardship, medical debt is a huge problem in the US. A Consumer Financial Protection Bureau study in 2017 found that 20 percent of Americans have at least one medical debt collection item in their credit reports, and that more than half of collection items on credit reports are for medical debts. Based on the most recent data from 2016, almost 40 percent of adults under the age of 65 reported that their credit scores were lower because of medical debt. This means they had trouble getting—or paid a higher interest rate on—home mortgages, credit cards and auto loans.

Those of us over 65 and enrolled in Medicare might think we are safe from ruinous medical costs, but this is not necessarily true. People incur out-of-pocket costs for medical care averaging $122,000 between the age of 70 and death. Those unlucky enough to have a serious illness (about 5 percent) will experience out-of-pocket costs of more than $300,000.

A poll taken by the *Associated Press* late in 2017 found that 48 percent of Americans named health care as the most important problem facing the country, far ahead of any other issue from taxes to immigration. A Reuters/Ipsos poll conducted in May/June 2018 found that 65 percent of Americans were "very concerned" about the overall cost of health care and that 66 percent of US adults were "concerned" about their ability to see a doctor of their choice going forward.

The United States was not always such a dramatic outlier. Back in 1980, US spending for health care was about 8.5 percent of our GDP— about the same as in Germany and the Netherlands. Spending in the other comparable countries clustered at around 6 to 7 percent of GDP. What has happened since 1980 is that we in the United States have spent more on activities that have no clinical benefit and do not improve the delivery of health care to our citizens, but do enrich the paper-pushers and hangers-on. Over the same period that our costs have ballooned relative to peer countries, our infant and child mortality statistics have gone from being roughly the same to significantly worse!

In many ways, doctors are almost as dissatisfied with the status quo as are patients. When I started my career, anyone talking about "burn-out" as a problem for physicians would have gotten a blank stare. Medicine was considered by most physicians to be a calling, and we felt privileged to be doctors. Physicians now increasingly feel caught between conflicting demands by patients, hospitals, regulators and insurers, all threatening to punish them for presumed transgressions of arcane rules. A headline story in a recent edition of the magazine

3

*Medical Economics* was "Why I Still Love My Profession." Apparently, enjoying the practice of medicine is now considered newsworthy!

I will explain why American healthcare is so expensive and suggest measures to cut costs dramatically while improving care.

Chapter 1

## Medicine Advances While Delivery Stagnates

Through much of human history, doctors had very few tools to change
the course of disease. Their role was more to comfort and advise than to
cure. This role has changed dramatically during my lifetime. The 1940s
saw the development of sulfa drugs and penicillin. Doctors could now
cure infections instead of simply hoping the body's natural defenses
would allow recovery. The 1950s saw the near elimination of the
scourge of polio through vaccination. A disease whose treatment
included iron lungs could now be prevented. In the 1960s surgeons
began to transplant organs. The 1970s gave us new forms of imaging—
CT and MR scanners and echocardiography—that allowed much earlier
and more precise diagnoses. Instead of having to open the body, doctors
could now see detailed pictures of internal organs.

When I was a resident, in the early 1970s, the standard approach to
Hodgkin's disease involved opening the abdomen and doing biopsies.
Now a non-invasive scan gives the treating doctor all the information
needed. The 1980s saw the rapid spread of angioplasty and stenting.
When I was a resident, our treatment of heart attacks was little different
than it had been for hundreds of years: we put the patients to bed and
watched them. We could use medicine to treat rhythm problems, but the
major "advance" in treating heart attacks was simply getting patients out
of bed sooner. Now when a patient comes to the Emergency department
with a heart attack, he or she is whisked off to the catheterization suite
and the blocked artery is opened. Typically, the patient can go home the
next day. In the twenty-first century, genomics is dramatically changing

the approach to inherited diseases and cancer. Many once-lethal diseases can be turned into chronic diseases—or even cured.

At the same time that we are witnessing these huge advances scientifically and technologically, we are also seeing costs spiral out of control. The early advances, such as antibiotics, gave us a very big "bang for the buck," with cures costing just a few dollars. Disease prevention through immunization has been very cost effective. Caring for a polio victim—pre-vaccine—involved long, expensive hospital and rehabilitation care. Preventing polio with a vaccine costs less than $100. Unfortunately, our more recent advances are much more expensive. The numerous, well-publicized high-tech advances that come with huge price tags have not increased life expectancy nearly as much as certain low-tech measures, such as decreasing the smoking rate. The new genomic-based treatments are often priced in the hundreds of thousands of dollars, or even millions. We are rapidly approaching the point when we will simply be unable to afford medical care.

The family doctor who oversaw your health care and treated most problems has given way to a vast array of specialists who tend to look at your health the way the blind men looked at the elephant. Hospitals that were looked on as charitable organizations have become huge profit centers. Medical advances are driven as much by Wall Street as by science.

As a practicing physician for almost 45 years, I have watched as our science became much more sophisticated and our ability to help patients vastly improved—while our system of delivering care deteriorated at an equally rapid pace. The lingering question is: what is wrong, and how can it be improved?

Chapter 2

## Why We Have the System We Do

Few countries tie health insurance as tightly to one's job as we do in the United States.

For most of our country's history, medical care was of limited benefit and medical expenses were low. After the discovery of penicillin and the dramatic explosion of new medications and technologies, medical care became both more useful and dramatically more expensive. Health insurance—designed to cover hospital and surgical care—began to be offered. The original Blue Cross plans were developed in the 1930s.

During World War II, labor was scarce with so many men sent overseas. A wage freeze prevented employers from attracting workers with higher wages, but benefits, including health insurance, were exempt. Employers began to dangle health insurance as a benefit to attract the best employees. Also, the Internal Revenue Service decided that employer contributions to health insurance premiums would be tax free, which meant workers paid less out of pocket. This system continues, and the US is unique among developed countries in tying most health insurance to employment. Roughly half of all Americans get their health insurance through their employer, while 19 percent are Medicare participants, 22 percent are insured through Medicaid, and 9 percent remain uninsured.

This coupling of health insurance to employment means that loss of a job means loss of health insurance, a double whammy if you must leave your job because of poor health.

Having an employer-based system also makes things particularly hard on small businesses. Small businesses have fewer insurance companies interested in selling them health insurance and tend to have higher costs for the health insurance that is available. If you are a General Motors, with tens of thousands of employees, a serious illness in one of your workers is unlikely to have a major impact on the overall health care spending of the entire group. However, if you own a boatyard employing 35 workers and one of your employees gets a serious illness and runs up big bills, you are likely to see your premiums sky rocket in ensuing years—if you can even find an insurer who wants to do business with you.

Since most newly-created jobs now come from small businesses, and because we are seeing increasing numbers of people employed in non-traditional employment situations such as contractors or nominally independent status (think Uber drivers), it is increasingly difficult for these workers to get any health insurance, or at least any they can afford.

There are also wide disparities in the percentage of workers who have health insurance based on occupation. Detailed surveys conducted in 2013 and 2014 showed that the percentage of workers 18 to 64 years old who did **not** have health insurance varied from 2 to 4 percent among occupations such as engineers, architects, teachers and librarians—to 37 to 38 percent among those working in fishing, farming, forestry, buildings and grounds, and maintenance. It is sad but not surprising that the workers in the most hazardous occupations, many of whom are self-employed or employed by small businesses, were least likely to have health insurance.

America stands alone among rich countries in not having essentially all its people covered by health insurance. There are many reasons for this, in addition to the accidental effect of World War II resulting in our employer-based system. America's strong culture of individualism plays a role. Many Republicans believe that health insurance is not a right but something people choose to buy or not buy in a marketplace, just as they choose to buy or not buy a new car or a fancier cell phone. The trouble with this analogy is that health care and health insurance are not like the typical consumer purchase. It is easy for most consumers to comparison shop for major purchases, and a broad choice is generally available. Moreover, if you decide money is tight this year, you can keep your old car for another year and still get to work. When you try shopping for health insurance as an individual, you may find that the few plans that are available are so expensive that you cannot afford them. Unlike cars or cell phones, the differences between different health insurance plans are extremely complicated and even a very sophisticated shopper may find the choices mind-boggling. Also, unlike most consumer purchases, health care, like food or shelter, is a critical need rather than a want.

Does it really matter whether or not you have health insurance? In many cases it makes a difference to your life and your health—as well as your wallet.

One sobering example is a case reported in the *American Journal of Tropical Medicine and Hygiene* in 2018. An American man with no health insurance travelled to West Africa without getting a pre-travel health consultation. He returned from Africa with a high fever and chills and sat at home feeling very sick while he waited for health insurance approval under the Affordable Care Act. His diagnosis—when he finally went to the hospital—was malaria, which he was lucky to survive.

A 1993 study found a 25 percent higher risk of death among uninsured adults compared with those who had private health insurance. The Institute of Medicine estimated in 2001 that 18,314 Americans between the ages of 25 and 64 died annually because of lack of health insurance. Another study, published in 2009, estimated that after adjusting for the differences between the insured and uninsured in obvious factors such as race, education, smoking status, etc., the death rate for the uninsured was still 40 percent higher. More recently, I found a study comparing the survival rates of patients under 65 with the disease follicular lymphoma, a form of cancer. The authors found that the death rate in patients without health insurance was double that of those with private insurance.

So, yes, having or not having health insurance is—for many people—a matter of life or death.

Chapter 3

It's the Prices, Stupid

When Bill Clinton was running for the presidency against George Bush, his campaign manager coined the phrase, "It's the economy, stupid," to convey the message that the single most important issue to voters was their pocketbooks. When looking at why we spend so much more on health care than other countries, we can easily say, "It's the prices, stupid."

Americans do not drive up the cost of health care in this country because we use so much of it. We do not "consume" more health care than do citizens of Canada or Europe. We do not see doctors more often or take more prescriptions, nor are we hospitalized more often—but we do pay a lot more for the same services.

In most European countries, notably Germany, people use many more services than Americans, but their national health bill is still much lower. The average American saw a doctor four times per year in 2011, compared to an average of 6.4 times a year in the rest of the OECD countries. In the United States in 2011, there were 131 hospital discharges per 1,000 people, while the OECD average was 160. Americans undergo more high-cost procedures such as joint replacements and coronary stents than does the average European or Canadian, but not a great deal more. In a recent year, 0.2 percent of Americans underwent total knee replacements, compared to 0.15 percent of Canadians and Europeans, but several high-income European countries, including Germany, Austria, Switzerland, Finland and Belgium, had comparable rates to those in the United States.

While some of our dramatic overall cost increases are due to a growing and aging population, a careful analysis published in 2017 showed that price increases were the dominant factor driving up our health costs. Although the US population is aging—and older individuals typically have more chronic illnesses and more health care needs than young people—the percentage of our population over 65 is less than it is in most OECD countries, and dramatically less than it is in Japan. Our aging population is not the reason our medical care costs are so much higher. Again, it is because we pay much more for the services we receive.

One example of how much higher our prices are compared to those in other countries is the cost of imaging. A family friend was vacationing in France when he developed severe back pain. Fearing a ruptured disk, he went to an outpatient radiology center and requested a CAT scan of his spine. He was billed the equivalent of $200 for the scan. In the United States, the national average price for the same scan, using similar equipment, was $1,450, with a range of prices from $750 to a staggering $10,200.

Another example is the cost of surgery. A different friend was in Paris when she fell and broke her hip. (Please note that France is not an especially dangerous country—it is just that many of our friends travel there.) She was admitted to a Paris hospital and had a hip replacement. Back at home in the United States, our friend's doctor confirmed that the surgery had been done well, and that it would have been done the same way in an American hospital. Her total bill for the hospitalization, surgery and physical therapy was the equivalent of $8,200. Had the surgery been done in the US, surgery and hospitalization would have cost $37,900, on average, with a range of $32,000-$45,000. Physical therapy would have been an additional cost.

Drug prices in the United States are also higher than anywhere else in the world. Many Americans have discovered they can save money by buying their prescriptions in Canada, though this is fraught with problems, including the fact that it is technically illegal.

American physicians earn approximately double what doctors earn in Europe. In 2017, a salary survey found that US doctors earned an average of $294,000 annually, with a marked discrepancy between primary care physicians at $212,000 and specialists at $316,000. The corresponding figures for other countries, as of 2016, in US dollars, is:

Canada: General practitioner $107,000; specialist $161,000
Switzerland: General practitioner $116,000; specialist $130,000
France: General practitioner $92,000; specialist $149,000
United Kingdom:  General practitioner $118,000; specialist $150,000

(It must be noted, and will be discussed in more detail in a later chapter, that the cost of medical education is dramatically higher in the United States than in any of the countries listed above.)

Chapter 4

## Who are the Villains?

When deciding why our health care costs are so high, there is plenty of blame to go around: health insurers, hospitals, doctors, lawyers, the pharmaceutical industry and Americans' lifestyle and behaviors all play a role in our current mess.

Health care is financially ruining the United States. The national debt is exploding and the biggest driver in our mounting deficits is health care expenditures. Federal Medicaid spending in 2008 was $201 billion and by 2016 this had ballooned to $389 billion. In the same year, Medicare spending reached $650 billion and accounted for 15 percent of the total federal budget. For the first time in US history, health care is the country's largest employer, having passed manufacturing in 2008 and the retail sector in December 2017. While politicians tout the growth in health care jobs in their home states as an economic win, they ignore the fact that these jobs with their associated costs are not good for the nation. Moreover, most of the growth has not come in the form of direct caregivers, who help sick people, but in the administrative jobs that add cost but do not help anyone feel better. While many of our hospitals are short of nurses, and home health agencies have trouble meeting the needs of their clients, administrative jobs in the health care sector have grown exponentially.

Demographics are not helping the problem. As we age, we tend to have more and more chronic diseases, and use more and more health care—and the US population is aging. According to the US Census Bureau, by 2030, one in every five US residents will be over 65, and by

2035 there will be 78 million people 65 or older compared to 76.4 million under 18. This aging of the population means that health care utilization will inevitably rise, which makes it even more critical that we begin now to rein in costs.

Where does the money go? The following chart gives a rough approximation:

| Sector/Product Expenditure | Percent of Health Care |
|---|---|
| Hospital Care | 32% |
| Physician services | 20% |
| Prescription medication (retail or administered) | 14% |
| Health insurers cost/profit | 12% |
| Home health care/nursing home | 8% |
| Dental care | 4% |
| Medical equipment/other services | 10% |

As with any complex issue, there is no one villain or single problem that offers a quick or simple painless fix. Our administrative costs are excessive. Hospitals in the US are much more expensive than those in other countries. We have too many specialists and not enough primary care doctors, and many of our doctors earn too much money. The malpractice environment in the US encourages excess testing and treatment. We pay more for medications than do people in any other country. Our lifestyles and habits contribute to excess illness and death. While reliable statistics are hard to come by, enormous amounts of money are wasted on needless tests and treatments—and on outright fraud.

Let us look carefully at each of these factors.

Chapter 5

## The Health Insurance Industry

Many years ago, while I was involved in developing the pre-hospital emergency medical care system in Massachusetts, I went with a group to meet with the then-President of Blue Cross Blue Shield of Massachusetts, John Larkin Thompson. We were ushered into a magnificent office, larger than any I had seen in the state offices or hospitals where I worked. I was taken aback to find that this was not Mr. Thompson's office, but that of his secretary! We were soon shown into the office of the Great Man himself, and one could barely see him at the far end of his office. Plush carpet made our approach to his desk soundless, and the furnishings would not have been out of place in the Presidential Suite at the Ritz. I realized, of course, that all of this was paid for by our health insurance premiums. I also realized that this magnificent suite of offices benefitted only its occupants. It certainly added no value for its subscribers.

The idea behind insurance is in essence a simple one: share risk among many people so that an illness or accident does not ruin any one person or family. The original health insurance cooperatives functioned in this way and were quite affordable. Insurance per se shares the risk but adds no value and should not carry a large overhead of its own—but in the United States it clearly does.

Current American health insurance companies have dramatically changed from their original intent. Many are investor-owned and have profit rather than public service as their driving force. Until the passage of the Affordable Care Act, millions of Americans were denied health insurance coverage because of "pre-existing conditions," which insurers applied very broadly at times. In some cases, insurers refused to insure very tall people, or people with a complicated family medical history or a hazardous occupation.

Health insurers are notorious for trying to "cherry pick" healthier people to enroll. I have noticed, as Medicare Advantage plans send me fliers, that a commonly touted benefit is discounted gym memberships. This is not of great interest to frail elders with multiple diseases, but it is a draw for the healthy elders the plans want to enroll. Insurance representatives are known to recruit seniors at square dances and other spots where healthy, active potential enrollees gather. I heard of a plan that had its enrollment center on the third floor of a building with no elevator. Only those who can climb two flights of stairs need apply!

The highest paid individuals in the current American health care system are the CEOs of our big health insurers. Six health insurance companies (Centene, Humana, Aetna, United Health, Anthem and Cigna) paid their CEOs more than $15 million in 2016. Smaller insurers pay their CEOs less, but the average insurance company CEO last year earned $584,000, far outstripping the average income of any other group working in the health care field.

While the direct cost attributed to health insurance companies is about 12 percent, the total costs attributed to our insurance system are more than double this figure. Administrative costs (i.e. billing and collection, claims review, prior authorization for tests and treatments, etc.) make up approximately 25 percent of the US health care bill, vastly higher than in any other country. The US has legions of people employed in the health care sector who add nothing of value to patients: medical coders, billing clerks, claims adjustors, drug purchasing agents, medical device brokers, etc. Duke University Hospital, with 900 beds, employs 1,500 billing clerks. The Montreal General Hospital, a teaching hospital of comparable size, employs fewer than 10. A study published in the *Journal of the American Medical Association* in February 2018 calculated that the cost to the doctor or hospital of billing and insurance-related activities ranged from $20.49 for a primary care visit (which is 15 percent of the total charge) to $215.10 for an inpatient surgical admission. While other industries typically employ 100 full-time-equivalents to collect $1 billion in goods or services, health care employs 770 full-time-equivalents to collect every $1 billion in physician services. The process of moving money from payers to hospitals and doctors consumes an estimated $50 billion annually.

In addition to collecting premiums and paying for charges, much of what insurance companies do, beyond managing their investment portfolios, is "make work" that does not help patients. Every doctor gets reams of faxes and emails pointing out things they already know about their patients, and often must spend time responding to these communications, an activity that adds to physician burn-out and rarely if ever helps their patients. Insurance companies have different requirements for submitting and processing claims, making it impossible for individual practices or hospitals to submit their bills efficiently. Insurers have different "formularies" that list which medicines they will pay for with lower patient co-pays, or even pay for at all. The differing formularies mean that doctors must choose between spending time up front figuring out which of several equivalent drugs they can prescribe for a patient, or spending time later dealing with phone calls from the pharmacy. The typical pharmacy call tells you that the medicine you prescribed will cost your patient $50 per month, while a nearly identical one will cost $25 per month. (Not to mention that formularies often change with the calendar, so that a preferred drug in December becomes a high co-pay drug in January and the process starts all over!)

Insurance companies are very skilled at erecting barriers to care, including pre-authorizations and denials of needed care, which require doctors and hospitals to spend time and money on paperwork that adds enormously to doctors' stress, but does not improve anyone's health. Very telling, and not a surprise to anyone on the front lines of care, was the recent news item about an Aetna medical director who admitted under oath that he rarely if ever reviewed patients' medical records before denying coverage of care. I have sat in my office and listened while my secretary answered numerous, pointless questions asked by a clerk with no medical background who is simply going down a lengthy and largely irrelevant checklist. A study found that 12.6 percent of physicians' charges are initially denied, but that 81 percent of these are later paid—but at the cost of enormous amounts of time spent by doctors and practice staff. An AMA survey in 2018 of 1,000 physicians found that 92 percent felt that prior authorization programs delay access to care, with 78 percent saying that prior authorization causes some patients to abandon recommended tests or treatments. Maddeningly, 30 percent said they had waited three or more days to get a decision from the insurance company. If these programs truly focused only on preventing unneeded tests, one could argue their benefit; but my experience is that expensive testing, whether indicated or not, is routinely denied. In all my years in practice, I almost never had a test or procedure that I strongly felt the patient needed refused in the end, but I often came close to throwing the telephone at the wall as I navigated the insurance bureaucracy to get approval. The underlying theory seems to be that if the process is made onerous enough, some physicians will give up trying and the insurance company will save money. Boston psychiatrist Elissa Ely had an Op-Ed piece in *The Boston Globe* that touched a nerve for most practitioners. She wanted to prescribe a drug for one of her patients that was "off-label," meaning it was not FDA-approved for the purpose she intended to use it for, but had ample data showing it worked. The out-of-pocket cost for this generic drug would have been $23 per month, too much for her indigent patient to afford. Dr. Ely spent many days and many phone calls navigating the insurance maze, and finally, miracle of miracles, was told the medical director (to whom she had not been allowed to speak) had approved its coverage. Since this was an "over-ride," the patient's co-pay for the medication would be $90 per month!

If a drug is very expensive, the insurer may simply refuse to pay for it. A recent study looked at the new class of drugs to treat chronic hepatitis C, a disease that can, if untreated, lead to liver failure and cancer of the liver. Highly effective drugs, which can cure hepatitis C in 95 percent of patients, became available in 2014 but are very expensive. The study found that coverage of the drugs was denied in 14.7 percent of Medicare recipients, 34.5 percent of Medicaid recipients and 52.4 percent of patients with commercial insurance!

Anthem Insurance in 2018 rolled out a policy telling subscribers that if an Emergency Department visit is not an emergency, they are fully responsible for the charges. Guess who decides whether a visit is an emergency? Asking patients to second guess an emergency is wrong. While some ED visits are clearly inappropriate even to a lay person (think common cold), others are not (think abdominal or chest pain). Patients should be able to err on the side of caution and not have to choose between their health and an unexpected, giant bill. I saw a wonderful example of this conundrum in a recent newspaper. The top half of the page had a story about Anthem's new policy, reporting that a man, who experienced sudden onset of severe back pain and went to the hospital ED on the advice of a neighbor in the medical field, was denied coverage for the visit because it was declared a "non-emergency" by Anthem. At the bottom of the same page, a public service announcement explained how to recognize a stroke by its key warning signs and urged the public to call 911 and go promptly to the emergency room if they observed any of these signs. The number one sign, posed as a question, was "Does the face look uneven?" Well, the most common cause of an "uneven" face as shown in the cartoon figure is not a stroke but Bell's palsy, a condition that should be seen promptly but which probably does not require an emergency room visit. As a physician, I can tell the difference between Bell's palsy and a stroke after I examine the patient; expecting a lay person to make this distinction is totally unreasonable.

Another expense that drives up the cost of insurance and adds nothing to anyone's health is the enormous amounts companies spend on advertising and sales, as each insurer tries to convince the public they are better than their competitors. Our mailbox, doubtless like yours, fills with glossy brochures from health insurers around open enrollment time, and we are invited to attend talks with refreshments by the same competing companies.

It is in vogue now for insurers to measure "quality." Both Medicare and most commercial insurance plans try to do this. They require doctors and hospitals to submit reams of data documenting that they do the things the insurance company has decided reflect quality care. While it is hard to argue against "quality," the problem is that while collecting all the data unquestionably costs a lot of time and money, there is no evidence that these efforts do anything to improve care. Moreover, no one seems to agree on what measures should be collected. A report in the journal *Health Affairs* found that in 2015, physicians in four common specialties spent $15.4 billion collecting and reporting "quality measures." A related survey of 23 health insurance companies found that they used a total of 546 different quality measures, few of which matched with those used by other insurers or with the 1,700 measures used by federal agencies. Most of the "quality measures" insurers request are things that can be quantified and reported, such as how often a patient getting a total knee replacement gets pre-operative antibiotics. The things that matter to patients, such as how well a patient is walking six months after surgery, are rarely looked at. It is not surprising that there is zero evidence that any of the insurers' "quality assurance" programs do anything that benefits patients in terms of their health.

Because doctors know they are being "graded" on how many of the boxes they check and are warned that failure to measure up may result in lower reimbursement or in being dropped from the insurance companies' lists, the need to compulsively meet these "requirements" all-too-often overrides the patient's agenda.

Health insurance companies that provide coverage for prescription drugs vary all over the map as to which medicines in a class they will cover, and even change their coverage when they find a better deal negotiated with the pharmaceutical industry. One of the things that made me pull out my hair was to have a patient tell me that the medicine they had been using successfully for years was no longer covered under their plan. We would then find a similar drug that was covered, get them on the right dose after some trial and error, only to have the patient come in over the winter and tell me that as of January 1, the new medicine would not be covered.

One of the problems with our mostly employer-based health insurance system is that the true cost of insurance is hidden from the recipients. Many perceive the cost to be the amount deducted from their paychecks, and feel the employer's share is "free" for them, not considering that money paid on their behalf for health insurance is money that could potentially be used by the employer for other benefits, or a higher salary. The cost for employer-sponsored PPO coverage for a family of four was calculated by Milliman as $25,826 in 2016, and is higher today. The employee's average cost, both premium contributions and out-of-pocket expenses, was calculated as $11,033. Some of the $14,000 plus that the employer paid could have been given to the employee in added salary or additional benefits if health insurance cost less. The mean cost of an employer-sponsored family health insurance policy is now more than 30 percent of the median family income! As part of a National Public Radio story on health costs, they interviewed the CEO of a small business in Pennsylvania, MCS Industries, which manufactures picture frames and mirrors. The CEO recounted that a decade earlier, an MCS family policy cost $1,000 per month and had no deductible. In 2018, a family policy cost more than $2,000 per month and carried a $6,000 deductible. Employers nation-wide are passing health care costs onto their employees by having them absorb a larger share of the insurance premiums and paying higher co-pays and deductibles. Data from the Bureau of Labor Statistics have shown that every time health insurance costs rise by one dollar, an employee's overall compensation is cut by 52 cents. Employers can only absorb so much. We have reached the point where even people with "good" insurance feel the financial pinch of health care

A more fundamental problem, apparently entrenched in the current system, is that health insurance has moved far away from the concept of insurance as the way to care for large expenses that are hard to anticipate and hard to pay. Imagine what auto insurance would cost if the policy paid for your gas, oil changes, new tires and routine maintenance. That is what health insurance has become. Routine check-ups, simple lab tests, office visits and relatively inexpensive medications are all billed to your health insurance. It costs the medical office just as much to bill for an inexpensive service as for a more expensive one. There is an equal administrative cost of billing your insurance plan for an inexpensive medication as for an expensive one. The proliferation of these charges adds to the cost of running a medical practice and ramps up the cost of care and insurance. If we paid out of pocket for the small ticket items and reserved insurance payments to cover such expensive items as hospitalizations, surgery and complex imaging, that money should in theory be returned easily in the form of lower insurance premiums.

Chapter 6

## The Hospital Industry

About 32 percent of US healthcare spending goes to hospital care.

If you cannot get a job as CEO of a health insurer, another good way to get rich in health care is to be CEO of a hospital. An analysis performed in 2017 for *The New York Times* by Compdata Surveys showed that the average hospital CEO was paid $386,000 and hospital administrators earned an average of $237,000, compared to $306,000 for surgeons and $185,000 for general physicians. Not surprisingly, large academic hospitals routinely pay their CEOs well over $1 million. At large hospitals there is a profusion of senior Vice Presidents and VPs of this and that, all earning six figure salaries and all needing secretaries and assistants. There is little or no "economy of scale" in health care. The ultimate transaction is one nurse and/or one physician with a patient. The larger the organization, the more layers of administration, with no added benefit to patients but with much higher costs.

I had first-hand experience with this in 1990, when five of us who worked closely together joined the Lahey Clinic as a primary care group. This was an era when "integrated systems" were popular and hospitals were gobbling up solo doctors and small practices. During the negotiations, I asked what seemed like an obvious question. Lahey administrators had told us that if we continued working at the same pace, we would earn the same income. "Since you are going to increase the overhead," I asked, "how are you not going to lose money on our practice?" The answer I got was basically, "Don't worry about it. We are business people and we understand these things." So, now that we were "Lahey Framingham," instead of solo practitioners, a well-paid practice manager, whose salary and benefits were added to our overhead, joined our staff. Our perfectly adequate phone system, now not considered up to Lahey standards, was replaced with a state-of-the-art system. Employee handbooks were produced. A portion of the costs of the Lahey Human Resources and other departments was added to our overhead. A year into this arrangement, the Lahey administration came to us complaining that they were losing money on our practice!

In most US cities where there is not a monopoly, with its associated freedom to charge more, you see duplication of services. Every hospital "has" to have its own CT and MR machines, even if only half that many are needed to serve the community adequately. It has been demonstrated repeatedly that surgeons and operating teams must perform a minimum number of complex surgeries to maintain their skills and get optimal patient outcomes. Nonetheless, you will frequently see multiple hospitals in one city doing open heart surgeries and other complex procedures at sub-optimal volume. Each hospital can proudly tout its full range of services, but the patient outcomes are not as good as they would be if the complex procedures were consolidated at fewer hospitals.

There are many ways that hospitals can "game" the system to increase their revenues. As one example, an obscure provision added to the Medicare Modernization Act of 2003 allowed hospitals where labor costs were higher than average to apply for increased Medicare payment rates. These Medicare waivers were granted under secrecy, and the granting of waivers did not always match the local cost of living. The hospitals that received waivers increased hiring, payroll, executive bonuses, technology use and lobbying. These investments did not improve patient outcomes, but they paid off for politicians. Lawmakers with a "waived" hospital in their district received a 22 percent increase in their total campaign contributions and a 65 percent increase in individual contributions from employees in their state's health care industry.

Hospital mergers and acquisitions have blossomed, and as competition is removed, monopoly pricing power goes up. In the 14 years between 1998 and 2012, the roughly 5,000 hospitals in the US saw 1,133 mergers and acquisitions. By comparison, in 2014 alone there were 1,318 deals and in 2015, 1,503 such deals. The advent of the Affordable Care Act, aka "Obamacare," with its influx of newly-insured patients, made the hospital business more attractive. Only insured patients can be counted on to be admitted and have their bills paid. While hospitals are notorious for hounding the uninsured for payment, they are not always successful at collecting the debts.

Hospital accounting would make Rube Goldberg proud. Every hospital has a "list price" for every service, but essentially no one pays these prices. Medicare pays a fixed amount for a given stay, based on the patient's discharge diagnosis. Not surprisingly, this gives hospitals a huge incentive to get Medicare patients out of the hospital as soon as they can justify a discharge, since they are paid the same whether the patient stays four days or 14. This has led to the often-observed phenomenon of discharging patients "quicker and sicker." Since they are often in no condition to go home, the usual next step is a nursing or rehab facility. Instead of a six-day hospital stay, the patient spends four days in the hospital and a week in a rehab facility. The hospital does better financially but the total cost to the system is higher, as the nursing home care charges are added to the cost of care.

Woe betide anyone admitted to a hospital who has some financial resources but no insurance. The hospital typically charges them "list price," even though this may be double or triple what Medicare or any commercial insurer would pay. If you are clearly indigent, the hospital will write off the charges and take credit for free care, but if you are a small business owner, you may find yourself in court battling these bloated charges.

Hospital bills are full of errors, almost always favoring the hospital, with charges for medications not given and tests not performed. An analysis by Medliminal Healthcare Solutions found that four out of five medical bills contain errors, many minor mistakes but others that result in overbilling patients by hundreds or thousands of dollars. There are duplicate charges for the same test or procedure, or charges for tests that were ordered but never done.

Hospitals are also notorious for marking up the prices of everything they use or give you. Think $5 aspirin! National Public Radio had a segment on a man who was protesting the price of his hip surgery. Among other issues, when he reviewed his hospital bill, he saw a

$26,068 charge for hardware. The maker of the hardware device, after many calls and emails, told him that the hospital would have paid about $1,500 for the device, a sum confirmed by the patient's surgeon.

As pressures mount for more reporting of "quality measures" of dubious value, often in different formats to different insurers, and as doctors are subjected to myriad other administrative demands, many physicians are selling their practices to hospitals and becoming salaried employees. Physician employment by hospitals grew 49 percent between 2012 and 2015. In July 2012, 26 percent of physicians were hospital employees and by July 2015, 38 percent were employed. Inevitably, the price of their services goes up as hospital overhead is added to the price. All insurers, including Medicare, will pay more to a hospital than to a private practice for the identical service. We see this over and over. A cardiology group gets paid, say, $800 for performing an echocardiogram in their office. The same echocardiogram, performed by the same technician using the same equipment at a hospital, now costs $1,920. The Medicare Payment Advisory Committee noted in its 2013 report that Medicare paid 141 percent more for a "level 2" echocardiogram in a hospital outpatient department relative to the same study performed in a physician's office. A study reported in 2017 concluded that when physicians were employed by hospitals, "this generates higher prices, higher spending and ambiguous changes in quality." There is no justification for paying much more for the same service simply because the label on the door has changed.

This discrepancy in payment has been used and abused in other ways. Some commercial testing lab owners have found it very profitable to buy up small struggling rural hospitals: they funnel tests through the hospital and get paid much more per test because the charge is coming from a hospital. An example is the 49-bed Chestatee Regional Hospital in Georgia, which had been for sale for some time when a lawyer named Aaron Durall bought it for $16 million in the summer of 2016. Mr. Durall also owned a lab in Florida, called Reliance Laboratories, that did high volume drug-testing. Following the purchase of the hospital, tests—even those performed at the Florida lab—were billed through Chestatee, and reimbursements were sky high. CBS News uncovered documents showing that Durall's lab made $67 million by billing tests through another rural hospital in Florida, and more than $31 million in eight months through a similar scheme with a small hospital in northern California. If, say, $14.40 is a fair price to pay a commercial lab for running a blood test, why should the same test, run on the same equipment, be reimbursed at $106 when done in a hospital?

While I have focused on the excessive costs of our hospitals, there are other serious issues that must be addressed. To give you the punchline first: if you can avoid a hospital stay you should do so. Hospitals are teeming with bad bugs—bacteria that are highly resistant to antibiotics—and these are easily spread from one patient to another. Basic hand-washing, shown by Dr. Ignaz Semmelweis 168 years ago to cut down on hospital infections, is still not practiced all the time in most hospitals. To recover from an illness or surgery, you need adequate sleep and good nutrition. In the typical hospital the food is bland and unappetizing, and malnutrition is a common problem in patients with long hospital stays, particularly the elderly. As for sleep, forget it—you are likely to be woken multiple times to have pulse and blood pressure checked, whether this is needed or not. Because it suits the hospital routine, the phlebotomist will likely visit you for a blood draw before the crack of dawn. Even a few days in bed make you more prone to blood clots and contribute to constipation, loss of muscle mass and loss of balance. Repeated blood sampling, often done "routinely" and of no benefit to you, can result in anemia. The problem is much worse in the Intensive Care Unit, where constant light and noise make day and night blend into one and contribute to disorientation, particularly among the elderly. These issues are well known and are not new, but there has been inadequate motivation for hospitals to change.

Chapter 7

## Stay Out of the Emergency Room!

While the emergency department (ED) is technically part of the hospital, ED visits have their unique problems. Many people have come to rely on the ED for much of their care, and the reasons for this vary. A family with two working parents may be unable to take time off to bring a child to a primary care physician (PCP), or they may not have a PCP. Often, medical issues arise outside of office hours. In many ways, the current emergency department is like the famous definition of home—it is where, when you show up, they have to take you in. Since ED care is much more expensive than seeing a doctor in his or her office, insurers tend to discourage ED visits, usually through very high co-pays. While this is a legitimate response to people who go to the ED for head colds or chronic back pain, it also places the burden of deciding what is a legitimate emergency on the patient, who is least able to make this decision. Is the pain in your chest a heart attack or gas? Even the emergency physician may not be able to tell until after completing tests.

Because emergency departments must be open 24 hours a day, seven days a week, they are inherently more expensive to maintain than a doctor's office or urgent care center open only during busy times. Even if few patients show up in the ED at 2 am, there must be adequate staffing on an 11 pm to 7 am shift to care for anyone who does come.

Another factor that drives up the cost of care in an ED is that, typically, the doctors who see patients in the emergency department know nothing about them and frequently have no access to their medical records. They may repeat tests recently done and, since they are also not able to offer follow-up, tend to over-test for all possible conditions. A trusted family doctor could focus on more likely problems and ask the patient to follow up by phone or in person if symptoms change.

ED visits are often over-billed. I learned this first hand when my son had some chest pain. We went to a small local hospital for a chest X-ray, and this showed a pneumothorax—a condition in which air escapes from the lung and compresses the lung—which needed surgical treatment. A chest surgeon agreed to meet us in the ED of the hospital where I worked and put in the needed chest tube. The surgeon completed the procedure with no intervention by any of the emergency physicians. After the procedure had been done, an ED physician poked his head in and asked my son how he was doing. "In a lot of pain" was the answer, and the physician prescribed some pain medicine. There was no other contact with this physician and my son was soon taken up to a room on the surgical floor. We later saw that the emergency physician group had billed for a "Level 5" comprehensive visit, a code intended to describe care given to complex and very sick patients needing comprehensive care from the emergency physicians. Nor was this an atypical happening. The advent of electronic medical records (EMRs) has made it temptingly easy for doctors, with a few clicks, to "write" a comprehensive visit that was not done. *The New York Times*, back in 2012, published a story entitled "Medicare bills rise as records turn electronic." They recounted the story of a health care consultant who went to the emergency room of a Virginia hospital because of a kidney stone. When he got the bill from the emergency room physician, his medical record, produced electronically, reflected a complete physical exam that the patient knew had never happened. The doctor described a complete exam of the lower extremities, but the patient said that he was wrapped in a blanket and that the doctor never even saw his legs. The doctor's group reduced his bill after he complained, but how many patients even think to complain?

Even if you are not treated, you may receive a bill! I have heard this tale from many of my patients and also had a personal experience. My other son was playing hockey when he got slammed into the boards and had severe back pain. A friend drove him to the emergency room at a large New Bedford hospital where he checked in at the desk and told them the problem. Two hours later he was still sitting in the waiting room, still in pain. He had not seen a doctor, had not had X-rays taken, and had not been given pain medication. He asked his friend to take him home, and he went to bed. A later outpatient X-ray confirmed that he had fractured one of his lower vertebra. Two weeks later he got a bill from the hospital for his emergency room visit! Only after several phone calls threatening to take this public did they agree to waive the charge for the "non-treatment."

Because they know that most patients coming into the ED are not choosing their physician and must see which ever physician is available, emergency physicians tend to charge significantly more than the insurance-allowed charges. They are aware that patients are going to come in whether or not the physician group has lower or higher charges. They do this to a much greater degree than do physicians in specialties where patients have the time to select their doctor. (Other specialties where the doctors know they are the only option do the same thing: anesthesiology, radiology and pathology round out the list of specialties that charge four or more times the Medicare-allowed fee, compared to the 1.6 to 1.8 times the allowed fee family practitioners charge.)

A potential financial nightmare occurs when you go for emergency care and later find out that the physicians treating you are not part of your health insurance company's "network." If you are seeing a specialist for an outpatient consultation, either you or your primary care doctor can find out if they are "in network," and if not select someone else. When you have an acute problem, you are generally forced to go to the closest facility. Even if you know that the hospital is one of your allowed facilities, you may later find out that the emergency physician group has opted not to join. They logically, from a self-interested viewpoint, decided that since most of their patients had no choice but to see them, they would not accept the negotiated lower fees and would charge what they want. I have had many patients over the years get socked with huge bills for this reason. They did nothing wrong—they went to the ED of the hospital covered by their insurance plan—and unknowingly accumulated hundreds or thousands of dollars in physician bills.

An article in *Health Affairs* in 2017 reported that 20 percent—or one in five—of emergency department visits can lead to surprise bills. They noted that in 2014, 20 percent of hospital inpatient admissions from the ED, 14 percent of outpatient ED visits, and 9 percent of elective inpatient admissions likely led to a surprise bill from out-of-network providers. A classic case was described on Vox.com on May 23, 2018. A 34-year-old man was attacked and left unconscious. Witnesses called 911 and the man ended up in an emergency department in downtown Austin, Texas. Told that his jaw was broken and that he would need surgery, he still had the presence of mind to get out his cell phone and verify that the hospital was in his insurance network. His reward for this diligence was a $7,924 bill from the on-call oral surgeon who repaired his jaw and who was **not** a network provider.

Chapter 8

Doctors

About 20 percent of health care spending goes to physicians.

Most experts agree that the backbone of a good health care system is an adequate supply of primary care physicians, and this is the general rule in most developed countries. I have long believed that continuity of care—a doctor and patient getting to know each other, the doctor being able to know how a patient's life situation and feelings would affect their willingness to follow a course of treatment—were important. This intuition has now been verified by a review the *British Medical Journal* published in June 2018. The authors found that increased continuity of care was associated with lower mortality rates! Despite the substantial technical advances in medicine, interpersonal factors remain important.

In most other countries, Internal Medicine and Pediatrics are considered specialty practice, and not primary care. Generalists are family practitioners. Even with this very narrow definition of primary care, 29 percent of physicians in the OECD countries are generalists. In Canada, 47 percent of physicians are generalists. In the US, even counting Internal Medicine and Pediatric specialists as primary care physicians still left only 33 percent of physicians in primary care, down from 50 percent in 1961. In fact, most Internists in the US are practicing in subspecialties of Internal Medicine (pulmonary disease, cardiology, kidney disease, etc.) and are not doing primary care. In the decade 1951-1960, 7 percent of physicians completing Internal Medicine residencies went into subspecialties. Between 2011 and 2015, 88 percent did!

Similarly, in 2002, 30 percent of pediatric residents became subspecialists and in 2015, 41 percent did.

Even in Boston, home to three medical schools and several world-class hospitals, finding a primary care physician is very difficult. I experienced this first hand when trying to find doctors for my patients as I contemplated retiring. Even with connections, I found almost no primary care doctors affiliated with academic hospitals who were willing to take on new patients. The lack of primary care doctors, and their increasing need to spend so much time on paperwork that their time with patients suffers, has spawned the "concierge" model of care. A "concierge" doctor greatly limits the number of patients under his or her care and promises longer appointments and more personal attention for a fixed monthly or annual fee, typically running $1,000 per year or more just for being accepted into their practice. If you want a doctor who will focus on YOU and not the computer, and who has the time to answer your questions and to see you promptly when you feel ill, you can find one, but at the cost of an up-front fee that may be thousands of dollars a year in some cities. What was once the norm has now become an expensive add-on. For the wealthy, this may be a cost worth paying, but for most Americans it is appealing but unaffordable.

Why do medical students, most of whom express an interest in primary care when they enter medical school, overwhelmingly choose specialty care over primary care? The answer is some combination of prestige, lifestyle and income. Students are often taught through their training period that subspecialty care is superior to primary care, and most of their teaching role models are specialists. The student loan debt carried by most graduating medical students is staggering—in the hundreds of thousands of dollars—and the higher incomes of specialty practice are a huge attraction.

In most European countries, the cost of medical school is nominal. The opposite is true in the United States. It may cost students upward of $10,000 just to apply to the average 10 schools to which aspiring doctors apply. The *US News and World Report* survey on higher education reported that for the 2017-2018 academic year, public medical schools charged in-state students an average of $34,700 for tuition and fees alone, while the average private medical school charged $54,877. Room and board are on top of this, of course. A survey showed that the average debt carried by a medical school graduate in 2010 was $161,739, and that by 2016 this had climbed to $179,000. 86 percent of graduates have at least some debt and 20 percent had student loan balances of more than $200,000. Graduating students know that picking a career in a specialty will allow them to earn much higher incomes. Also, most specialties allow much more attractive work schedules than does primary care, and some lucrative specialties such as dermatology and ophthalmology allow a weekday nine to five schedule while still providing a high income.

The old saying has it that "if the only tool you have is a hammer, everything looks like a nail." If you are skilled at putting scopes down peoples' esophagus and if you are very well paid to do so, then a patient coming to you with heartburn is very likely to have endoscopy performed, followed by a prescription medicine to reduce acid. If the same patient were to go to their primary care doctor with uncomplicated heartburn, they are much more likely to be prescribed acid suppressing medication without a "scope." In the end, the result of seeing a primary care physician or a gastroenterologist will be the same, but in specialist hands, the cost will be thousands of dollars more. You may think that having an endoscopy is safe and that by having it nothing serious is missed, but sedation must be used to perform the test, and is far from risk free. Joan Rivers died from sedated endoscopy! The best estimate is that there is one death in 9,000 procedures—a rare event to be sure—but since about 18 million sedated upper and lower endoscopies are done annually in the United States, "routine endoscopies" may cause 2,000 deaths annually.

Throughout the world, specialists tend to earn more than generalists, but the discrepancy is higher in the United States, where specialists earn an average of 50 percent more. Why are specialists' incomes so much higher? A major role is played by the little-known and secretive Relative Value Scale Update Committee that sets Medicare fees, which are in turn generally used by commercial insurance companies to set their own higher fees. Specialists dominate this powerful body, and in the spirit of "you scratch my back and I will scratch yours," fees for procedures are set much higher than fees for sitting down with patients and examining and advising them. Fees for innovative new procedures are set particularly high, and rarely do these come down when the procedure is in common use. The time-consuming process of getting to know a patient and establishing rapport is essentially valueless in this brave new world, because it is not a "billable procedure."

You may think, "But don't I get better care from a specialist?" Not necessarily. A widely reported study published in the journal *JAMA Internal Medicine* in 2018 looked at death rates for high risk patients with heart attacks or congestive heart failure admitted to teaching hospitals. They compared death rates during the period when major national cardiology meetings were held and the times before and after these meetings. The meetings attract thousands of cardiologists, including many from the teaching hospitals. The authors expected to see a surge in death rates when fewer senior cardiologists were working, but found the opposite—that death rates were lower! While this does not prove that having specialists around increases death rates, it certainly does not show that specialist care is better.

Over-billing by doctors is a common problem. In Massachusetts, a routine eye exam is covered by many insurers with no co-pay or need for a referral from the primary care physician. Since this visit is paid at a lower level than a problem-focused visit, ophthalmologists try to turn every routine eye exam into a "sick visit." I experienced this when I went for an exam with no complaints about my eyes. The examining doctor commented that I had early cataracts. I noted that this was perfectly normal for my age, just as was my graying hair, and that this was not bothering me at all. Months later I got the bill and found that my routine eye exam was now coded as a visit for cataracts and had been rejected by my insurance company because of a lack of referral. It took me months and numerous phone calls to get this resolved. In my practice, virtually every patient who scheduled a routine eye exam resulted in a call to my office from the ophthalmologist's office asking for a referral for some vague "problem," so that the ophthalmologist could bill at a higher rate.

Because doctors are typically paid much more to do a procedure than to talk to and examine patients, the temptation is always to do more procedures. If a dermatologist is quite sure that a skin lesion is harmless, he or she can reassure the patient of this and charge, say, $68.40 for a consultation; or they can biopsy the lesion to be even more certain and charge $280. Which are they more likely to do?

One of my patients came in very upset because her gynecologist of many decades had announced that now that the patient had turned 65 and gone on Medicare, she would no longer see her because she did not take Medicare! I can accept, grudgingly, that a doctor has the right not to see new Medicare patients because of the lower fees paid compared to commercial insurance, but I could never accept that a doctor would refuse to see a patient of long standing because they would get a reduced fee. What was once a sacred bond has, all-too-often, become simply a commercial transaction.

Just as this book was going to press, New York University made a blockbuster announcement: starting with the 2018-2019 academic year, medical school will be tuition-free for all students. To date, no other schools have announced plans to do the same, and NYU was able to do this because of generous donations to their permanent endowment fund. This will be a fascinating, real-world experiment to watch. One hopes that this development will allow the school to accept more minority and other disadvantaged students who are now deterred by the high cost of medical school. Another hope is that allowing students to graduate without a mountain of student loan debt will encourage them to go into primary care or practice in communities where they are most needed. If this happens, we will have a model for how medical schools should be run. If there is minimal change in student choices after graduation, it will suggest that financial aid will need to be more targeted to encourage these behaviors.

Doctors undergo a long period of education and post-graduate training, and often work under stressful conditions. They are entitled to be paid comparably to professionals who perform similarly highly skilled work. There is, however, no reason why any physician needs to earn much more.

Chapter 9

Lawyers

On a sunny morning in May 2018, I sat in a conference room in a law office in downtown Boston, surrounded by six lawyers and a stenographer. The lawyers had all flown in from half-way across the country to take my deposition as an expert witness in a malpractice case. I had one overwhelming thought: "What an enormous waste!" The case involved a man in his forties who had gone to the emergency department of a major hospital with the sudden onset of chest pain. He was discharged less than 24 hours later, still having pain and with an erroneous diagnosis. He saw his family doctor the next day, who advised him to continue the medications given by the hospitalists. That night he died, and he was found at autopsy to have been suffering from an aortic dissection.

While surgery has significant risk, prompt diagnosis and surgery might well have saved his life. All four of the doctors involved in his care were now being sued. Each doctor had his own lawyer, now present in the room. There was also a lawyer representing the hospital and a lawyer representing the law firm that had engaged me. Each of the six lawyers was billing for one to two days of their time, plus airfare, hotel and meal expenses, all of which would come out of any settlement. Why could not the hospital and doctors have gone to the widow and said they were truly sorry; that the condition was not common but could have been diagnosed; that surgery was high risk but should have been done; and that they wanted to compensate her and try to ensure that if a similar patient came in, the staff would be better trained to recognize it?

Malpractice insurance is a substantial cost of operating a medical practice. In Massachusetts, the annual cost for a standard $1 million/$3 million policy (which covers up to $1 million per claim and $3 million per year) ranges from a low of $7,382 for psychiatrists; to $11,836 for family practice with no surgery; to $36,225 for general surgery; to a whopping $68,230 per year for obstetrics and gynecology with major surgery. This cost is obviously built into the expenses that doctors must cover in their charges.

The "at fault" litigation-oriented malpractice system in the United States is good for lawyers but bad for doctors and patients. The system takes much too long to conclude—two to four years if the case goes to trial—and siphons off too much money to lawyers. The result of a malpractice suit often hinges on how sad a case can be presented to a jury rather than the degree of fault. Bad doctors with engaging personalities often cause repeated harm without getting sued, while conscientious doctors who take on difficult cases, and do their best, may pay out because of a bad outcome rather than bad practice. Given the usual contingency fee arrangement, lawyers are reluctant to take on cases where there is clear malpractice if they anticipate a low payout. An acquaintance of ours had his bladder punctured by an improperly placed catheter, missed work while it healed and wanted to sue for lost wages. No lawyer would touch his case because their share of his anticipated payment was too low to be worth their time. It would have been much easier to find a lawyer willing to take his case had he been looking for a large award for "pain and suffering."

Every doctor readily admits to ordering more tests than are indicated due to fear of being sued because they missed something. The exact contribution of this to excessive testing is hard to quantify with certainty, but it is real and substantial. A study published in the *Archives of Internal Medicine* in 2010 found that 90 percent of 1,231 physicians surveyed said that doctors order more tests than medically needed to protect themselves from lawsuits, and a similar survey conducted in 2017 found that fear of malpractice suits was the leading cause of unnecessary testing, cited by 85 percent of doctors. Several studies published between 2003 and 2013, quoted by Berlin, estimated the cost of "defensive medicine" to be anywhere from $56 to $162 billion annually. "Hard" data quantifying the role that fear of malpractice plays in over-testing and over-treating has been difficult to get, but a study published in June 2018 in *JAMA Cardiology* provides some insights. Patients with chest pain can have a variety of tests—ranging from a good history and physical, to stress testing and even to a coronary angiogram—to help the doctors decide if the pain is heart-related. Each step "up" the testing ladder adds both costs and risks. The research team looked at how doctors approached such patients, comparing those in states with newly-installed caps on malpractice payments to those in states without such caps. The doctors practicing in states with caps on malpractice ordered 24 percent fewer angiograms as the first test than did doctors in states without such caps—saving substantial money and subjecting patients to less risk. Another study published in July 2018 by the *National Bureau of Economic Research* looked at testing in military hospitals, where the doctors are shielded from malpractice suits by active duty personnel but not by dependents treated at the same hospitals. They estimated that when there was no threat of lawsuits, there was 5 percent less testing and no evident harm from less testing.

Doing unnecessary tests not only costs considerable money, but it is often misleading. The best example is advanced imaging (CAT scans and MRIs) for back pain. Virtually every guideline says that for acute low back pain, in the absence of "red flags" such as suspicious clinical findings, there is no need to do such imaging. None the less, they are commonly ordered, primarily because of patient insistence and fear of lawsuits, should something be missed. Because the large majority of middle aged and older adults—even those who never have had a backache in their life—have some abnormality on an image of the back, the test will show some abnormality. This may lead to a referral to a back specialist, who may then suggest surgery to "fix the abnormality." Since the back pain was muscular or arthritic, and the "abnormality" had nothing to do with the pain, the patient will almost never be helped, but may often be made worse.

The adversarial system inherent in the current malpractice environment also discourages doctors and nurses from reporting an adverse event that they hope might go unnoticed, or from reporting "near misses" from which the system might learn and improve. Every doctor, even the best, makes mistakes. Good doctors learn from their mistakes. In a less litigious world, all adverse events and near-misses would be reported and discussed, and staff could learn from these mistakes, making them less likely to recur. There is, however, little incentive to discuss something that might lead to system improvements if you fear that doing so may expose you to a lawsuit.

Chapter 10

## The Pharmaceutical Industry

While spending on medication makes up only about 14 percent of total US health care spending, it is dramatically increasing and represents one of the most egregious failures of a "free market system" to be reasonable and fair. A 2018 report from the National Academy of Science concluded that "consumer access to effective and affordable medicines is an imperative for public health, social equity and economic development; however, this imperative is not being adequately served by the biopharmaceutical sector today." In 1960, the outpatient prescription drug market was $2.7 billion and 96 percent of the cost was out of pocket. By 2017, the estimated market for outpatient prescription drugs had ballooned to $360 billion, only 13 percent of which was paid out of pocket. US pharmaceutical expenditures last year were $1,443 per capita. In Germany the comparable figure was $667 per capita; in the Netherlands it was $656; and in Sweden $566. Americans do not use more medications but they do pay a lot more for them. The biopharmaceutical industry has the highest profit margin of any sector of the economy.

"Jack" (not his real name) was one of my favorite patients. He had a heart as big as his very large body, and had spent years caring for his ailing mother and later his girlfriend who was sick with cancer. After they both died, his companion was his dog, for whom he cared deeply. Jack was diabetic, and his diabetes was not well controlled despite my increasing his insulin dose. At one visit I asked Jack if he was taking the insulin twice daily as prescribed. He admitted that he was only taking it once. The reason? Despite having health insurance through his company, his co-pay for the insulin was so high that he told me, "it is either take the full dose or feed my dog." No one should have to make that choice, nor the choice between medicine and heating oil that hits many seniors in the winter, nor between medicine or new clothes for the children.

It was particularly ironic that Jack was having trouble paying for his insulin. Insulin was discovered by Canadian doctors Frederick Banting and Charles Best in 1921, and they sold the patent to the University of Toronto for $1, believing that a drug this important and life-saving for diabetics should always be available and affordable for those who needed it. Drs. Banting and Best would be spinning in their graves if they knew how Big Pharma was handling their discovery.

Drug prices in Canada are dramatically lower than those in the United States for the same medications. As of February 2018, the average wholesale prices for a few randomly selected drugs were:

| Apixaban (Eliquis) | US $419 | Canada $101 |
| Epinephrine injection (EpiPen) | US $608 | Canada $189 |
| Insulin glargine (Lantus) | US $77 | Canada $20 |
| Rosuvastatin (Crestor) | US $261 | Canada $55 |
| Sitagliptin (Januvia) | US $430 | Canada $96 |

Unfortunately for American patients, importing drugs from Canada is illegal. Even if this law is not always enforced, many pharmacies claiming to be reselling Canadian medications are selling drugs that were manufactured elsewhere, often in China or in India, that may or may not be of comparable quality.

I mention Canada because it is our next-door neighbor, and because many of my patients had begun trying to buy their prescription medicines there, but I could use virtually any other country in the world for a comparison. Five pens of Tresiba, a new form of insulin, cost about $500 at retail in the United States. In Spain, the same box of five pens costs five Euros—about $6. A vial of antivenom, used to treat rattlesnake bites, was billed to patients in Arizona at between $7,900 and $39,652 per vial a couple of years ago, while a very similar product produced in Mexico retailed in that country for $100.

A congressional report released in March 2018 reported that the prices of the 20 most commonly prescribed brand-name drugs for seniors have risen nearly 10 times more than general inflation over the past five years. Twelve of the 20 drugs saw their prices increase by more than 50 percent over the five-year period, and six had prices increases of more than 100 percent.

"Ruth," not her real name, was a sweet independent lady in her eighties who was remarkably well but troubled by urinary urgency. We tried several older medications that were affordable but did not help her problem very much. I gave her samples of a newer medicine that she found quite useful, but when I gave her a prescription, I got a phone call the next day. "Doctor, did you know they want over $400 a month for that medicine?" She concluded that she would rather live with her problem than pay half her Social Security check for one prescription.

Why do we pay so much in this country?

The poster child of greed in the pharmaceutical industry is Martin Shkreli, former CEO of Turing Pharmaceuticals (now renamed Vyera Pharmaceuticals). In August 2015, Turing bought up the patent for Daraprim, a drug first created back in 1952 that was life-saving for patients with severe toxoplasmosis. Toxoplasmosis is a common infection that rarely causes symptoms except in people with weakened immune systems or in pregnant women. In these groups it can cause encephalitis (brain infection), retinal infection leading to blindness or miscarriage. Treatment for these conditions is mandatory and Daraprim is the only available drug that works.

Turing quickly boosted the price of the drug by 5000 percent— from $13.50 per pill to $750 per pill. A course of treatment costs $45,000 a month, and a typical course of treatment lasts at least six weeks. The manufacturer was called in front of congressional panels to answer questions about the price increase, but the price never came down. Nor was this an isolated event. Cycloserine, a drug used to treat dangerous multidrug-resistant tuberculosis, was increased in price from $500 to $10,800 for 30 pills after its acquisition by Rodelis Therapeutics in 2015. In 2010, Valeant acquired the rights to Syprine, a drug invented in the 1960s to treat Wilson's disease, a very rare disease that I never saw in 45 years of practice. Valeant raised the price by more than 3000 percent, from $652 to $21,267 per month. Less dramatically, a widely used antibiotic, doxycycline, went from $20 for a 10-day course of treatment in October 2013 to an average of $185 a bottle in April 2014. More recently, the price of an Epi-Pen (injectable epinephrine), a critical life-saving drug used to treat severe allergies, was dramatically raised. Mylan Pharmaceutical bought the rights to the drug in 2007, when a two-pack cost about $100; by 2016 the same two-pack cost more than $600. Meanwhile, Mylan's CEO, Heather Bresch, saw her pay go from $8 million in 2012 to $18 million in 2015.

The astute reader may ask why, since these were all generic drugs, long past any patent protection, did another manufacturer not step up and compete. In the case of Daraprim, Cycloserine and Syprine, the underlying reason was the rarity of the diseases they treated. Only about 6,000 patients in the US annually require treatment for toxoplasmosis, and Wilson's disease occurs in about one in 30,000 people. Generic manufacturers knew that if they geared up to make the drugs and spent the $200,000 or so needed to go through the regulatory process, the original manufacturer could simply cut prices dramatically and not allow them to make a profit. According to Sanofi-Aventis, which markets an injectable epinephrine competing with Epi-Pen, Mylan created multiple barriers to prevent Sanofi's drug from getting market share. These, they say, included "new and unprecedented rebates" to insurance companies and pharmacy benefit managers, with the condition that they refuse to stock Sanofi's product.

In some instances the US government, specifically the Food and Drug Administration (FDA), has contributed to the problem. Many old drugs antedated the FDA and were grandfathered in for marketing as cheap generic medications. In 2006, the FDA started a program to allow pharmaceutical companies limited monopolies if they did the safety and efficacy testing now required for new drugs, on these older drugs. This can bring big paydays for the producers. A wonderful example is colchicine, a drug known to the ancient Greeks for its efficacy in treating acute gout. Through most of my career, it generally cost about 25 cents a pill. URL Pharma, the small Philadelphia drug maker granted rights over colchicine after they ran some small clinical trials and proved that colchicine worked to treat gout, was bought by Takeda Pharmaceuticals for $800 million in 2012. Asia's biggest drug maker has since brought in $1.2 billion in revenue from the branded drug, sold as Colcrys, which went on the market at a wholesale price of almost $6 a pill. Takeda says testing for FDA approval made the drug safer. In fact, there was so much experience with the drug that it was a "no-brainer" that testing would show that the drug was effective. Many of my long-term gout patients became apoplectic when they refilled their prescriptions after this FDA-mandated "advance."

Many different forms of synthetic cortisone are available, most of which are more or less the same. Not all are sold in all countries, but since they are equivalent, this is not a serious issue. One that has been sold in Europe, but not in the United States, and is effective in treating Duchenne muscular dystrophy is deflazacort. Duchenne muscular dystrophy, a rare inherited disease that has no cure, occurs in about one out of every 7250 male babies. It causes progressive muscle weakness, eventually affecting the heart and the muscles that allow breathing, and leads to death by age 30. For many years, both deflazacort and the more well-known similar synthetic cortisone, prednisone, have been used to slow the progression of the disease, even though they were not officially labelled for such use. The effectiveness of both drugs is similar, though deflazacort causes a bit less weight gain. If the treating doctor wanted his or her patient to use deflazacort, it was available from Europe at a cost of about $2000 per year. (The FDA does allow importation of drugs under specific conditions, including unavailability commercially in the US.) In 2017, the FDA granted approval for deflazacort to be labelled for use to slow the progression of weakness in Duchenne dystrophy. Marathon Pharmaceuticals had purchased the rights to sell the drug in the US and priced it at $89,000 a year—44.5 times the prior price for the drug imported from Europe! Moreover, since there was now commercial availability in this country, importation became illegal. Even though the drug is generic, because Duchenne dystrophy is a rare "orphan" disease, the manufacturer was allowed a seven-year exclusive right to sell. No benefit to patients or their families but much higher cost and big bucks for big pharma.

In the category of "How could this possibly be?" is the story of an old timer called Acthar gel. This is an injectable form of ACTH, a hormone that stimulates the adrenal glands to make more cortisone. As such, it has very little advantage in effectiveness or safety over the widely available and still relatively cheap drug prednisone, a synthetic form of cortisone. Acthar gel was approved by the FDA in 1952 for infantile spasms, for which there is modest evidence that it helps, and for a variety of rheumatic diseases and sudden worsening of multiple sclerosis. For the latter conditions, the evidence that Acthar gel helps is very limited, and the small studies supporting its use were mostly conducted by researchers with strong ties to the manufacturer. Despite this very limited data for benefit, aggressive marketing by the manufacturer has led to continued use of Acthar gel, notably for multiple sclerosis, despite its growing price tag. A vial of the drug increased in price from $1,650 to more than $24,000 when Questcor bought the patent in 2001, and continued to rise. Mallinckrodt acquired the patent in 2014 and the price increased again, and as of 2017 the price was $34,000 per vial. Between 2011 and 2015 Medicare spent $1.3 billion on a drug of very little benefit that probably should not even be on the market. A recent CNN exposé discovered that more than 80 percent of doctors who filed Medicare claims for injecting Acthar gel in 2016 had received money or other perks from the manufacturer. Between 2013 and 2016, Questcor and Malinckkrodt paid more than $6.5 million for speaker fees and "consultations" to doctors who used their drug.

Across the board, brand name drug prices rise relentlessly, by about 15 percent a year, far outstripping inflation. In most developed countries, single payer health systems use their clout to negotiate big discounts, and in some cases refuse to let a drug be marketed if its cost is not justified by its value. Most new products released by the industry are simply minor variations on an existing product, on which they then spend huge amounts of money marketing what I call "me too" drugs. A wonderful example is in the acid-suppression class. When omeprazole (Prilosec) was introduced, it was a real improvement in treating ulcers and heartburn, and became very profitable for its manufacturer, Astra Zeneca. Other pharmaceutical companies developed similar products, which were not any better except in the eyes of their detail reps (pharmaceutical company employees who call on doctors to tout the wonders of their company's products). When the patent on Prilosec ran out, Astra Zeneca made a minor tweak in the molecule and introduced esomeprazole, branded as Nexium, "the new purple pill," and tried hard to get doctors to use this preferentially over the now generic omeprazole. In a country with a central purchasing authority, Astra Zeneca would be told, "OK, you are welcome to sell Nexium, but only if it is priced competitively with omeprazole." In the US, every health plan must negotiate separately. Astra Zeneca is free to price Nexium at five times the cost of omeprazole and blanket the airways to convince doctors and the public that it is better. Medicare, the largest single payer for health care in the US, is specifically barred by law from negotiating drug prices.

The drug companies try to justify their sky-high prices based on the need to cover their high costs of research and development. This argument has several holes in it. The first is that while they do spend considerable money on R+D, they spend even more on marketing. Over the past decade, pharmaceutical companies spent almost twice as much on marketing and administrative costs as on R+D. If they spent less money marketing, they would be able to shift some of this money to R+D. I could more easily accept this argument if all their research went into developing innovative medications that solved a problem, but the majority of their research goes into developing "me too" drugs. One company comes out with a truly innovative product that gives doctors and patients a better medication; other companies then spend their resources tweaking the original molecule so they can sell a similar product, on which they then spend even more money marketing it as better than the original. Numerous examples abound. The first ACE inhibitor (angiotensin converting enzyme inhibitor) developed was captopril, patented in 1975 and approved for marketing in the US in 1981. This medicine proved very useful in treating high blood pressure and later in treating congestive heart failure. It was followed to market two years later by enalapril, and there are now 10 ACE inhibitors on the market, all with similar benefits and similar side effects. All the branded products are expensive. Why compete on price? The leading side effect of ACE inhibitors is an annoying (though generally harmless) cough. A new class of medications, called ARBs (angiotensin receptor blockers) have most of the benefits of the ACE inhibitors but do not cause a cough. The first in its class to be useful for routine use was losartan, which was approved for marketing in 1995 after considerable R+D work. In 2018, we now have seven ARBs on the market with more on the way, all essentially the same. I could fill pages with other examples, but you get the idea. A truly innovative product should make a decent profit for its developer, but why should companies be equally rewarded for selling an essentially similar product that is competing based primarily on marketing?

New cancer drugs now routinely come to market with price tags of more than $100,000, and $400,000 is becoming the new norm. Such a price tag might be justified for a drug that makes a dramatic difference in length and quality of life, but many of these "blockbuster" drugs add only marginal improvement over existing therapies, yet carry the same outrageous price tags. One example is neratinib, approved in 2017 for patients with early stage breast cancer. A study showed that it improved invasive-disease-free survival after two years follow-up by 2 percent—from 92 percent to 94 percent (without any published data showing improved overall survival). This marginal benefit from a drug with a cost of $10,500 per month! The FDA can "fast-track" so called breakthrough drugs that promise to help serious conditions such as cancer and life-threatening infections. The evidence supporting the usefulness of these drugs is often very flimsy, based on small, poorly-designed trials and often using surrogate outcomes. (Surrogate outcomes are things like improvement in lab tests rather than prolonging life or making patients feel better.)

The drug companies claim that their prices are justified because of a widely-accepted study, first published in 1979 and last updated in 2014, which estimated it took 10 years and $2.7 billion to develop a single drug. Critics of the industry repeatedly have questioned this study, done by Tufts Medical School but funded by the pharmaceutical industry, as its underlying data has been kept as a "trade secret" and has not been made available for analysis. In November 2017, researchers used the Securities and Exchange Commission's mandatory filings by start-up companies to study the true cost of new drug development. They found that the actual cost of developing a new drug is about one fourth of that claimed by the industry-sponsored study! A wonderful example of the disproportion between development costs and profits is found in the recently-approved sofosbuvir (brand name Sovaldi) used to treat hepatitis C. This was developed by a start-up biotech firm called Pharmasset, which spent $315 million on research over 12 years. Gilead Science bought the company and its promising drug in 2011 to for $11 billion! In the first quarter of 2017 alone, Gilead sold $2.6 billion worth of sofosbuvir, dwarfing its development cost.

Pharmaceutical companies rarely acknowledge the enormous amount of public funding that indirectly helps them. An analysis of the 210 new drugs the FDA approved between 2010 and 2016 found that the NIH provided funding of the basic research for each one.

Not satisfied with exorbitant prices, the pharmaceutical industry works hard to increase demand for its products. Among Western countries, only the US and New Zealand permit direct-to-consumer drug advertising. I had a wonderful cartoon in my office, showing a patient sitting on an exam table and the doctor asking, "How are you feeling?" In the next panel, the patient, pulling out a long sheet of paper, says, "I feel fine, but I have a list of things the drug companies said I should ask about." I am not much of a TV watcher, but when I spend an hour watching television, I must see five to 10 ads for medications. These are very stereotypic. An actor, playing a patient with a disease, is morose and blue, lamenting his inability to spend time with family or do other things he enjoys. His doctor prescribes the new magic pill, and now he is happy and smiling, doing everything he previously could not do. A long (and mandatory) recital of the horrid side effects the drug can cause is buried beneath the prior visuals. These ads must work, or the drug companies would not spend the money to run them. But when you listen to the hair-raising list of side effects, you wonder why anyone would ever take them! An article in the *Los Angeles Times* in February 2017 reported that drug companies spend more than $5 billion per year pitching prescription medications directly to the public.

The drug companies also work very hard to get doctors to prescribe their products. In the not-too-distant past, their attempts were blatant bribery. Doctors were offered all-expense-paid trips to resorts to hear "educational seminars" extolling the sponsoring company's products. Dinners at expensive restaurants, spouse included, were another opportunity to hear a sales pitch. With the adoption of a new code of conduct, these flagrant events are much less common, but doctors who want to eat out without their spouses can still do so just about every night. The ubiquitous detail person, who shows up in doctors' offices with lunch, samples and glossy brochures, is not there to provide objective information. Despite doctors' protestations that they cannot be bought by a free lunch, there is ample data to show that such visits do influence prescribing habits. A recent study published in *JAMA Internal Medicine* found that cancer doctors who had received any payments from pharmaceutical companies were 80 percent more likely to prescribe a cancer drug from that company than a drug in the same class from another company, when compared to specialists who had not received any such payments. The researchers were able to neatly graph numbers of meals received against numbers of prescriptions written, and found that the more meals, the more prescriptions! A CNN report dated July 27, 2018, reported that Bayer paid doctors millions of dollars in speaking and consulting fees to encourage the use of their implantable birth control device, Essure.

Marketing costs were particularly high for a small Arizona-based company called INSYS Therapeutics, which manufactures Subsys. Subsys is a form of the highly potent narcotic fentanyl, which can be used as a spray under the tongue for fast absorption. It was approved for use by cancer patients whose pain is uncontrolled with other narcotics, but company reps pushed it for any severe pain. Marketing costs for opioid-related drugs by Teva and Janssen, the second and third highest reported, were $869,000 and $854,000 in 2015. The marketing expenses of INSYS were $4,538,000! Not surprisingly, INSYS was accused in a whistle-blower suit of offering kickbacks to doctors who prescribed its product.

There is also the attractiveness factor. As my wife has pointed out, most "detail reps" are attractive young people. Twenty years ago, when most doctors were still male, these were attractive young women. As more women enter the profession, gender equality has followed in the ranks of drug reps, but being attractive and personable is still the rule.

Even more of a concern to me than the excessive "detailing" of medications to practitioners is that many medical thought leaders and academics are heavily subsidized by the pharmaceutical industry. These are the "experts" who, for one example, arbitrarily lowered the blood sugar level at which diabetes should be diagnosed. This instantly created millions of more diabetics—and potential customers for diabetic medications! Specialty societies typically convene expert panels to recommend best practices, which good doctors are expected to follow. If you look carefully, many, if not most, of the members of these panels receive research funding and hefty speaker fees from big pharma. It is hard to believe that these professors are really giving unbiased advice when they are receiving four-figure fees and generous travel expenses to give a lecture, or when much of the budget for their research is coming from the drug companies.

Another blatant conflict of interest, detailed in a story in *Science* magazine in July 2018, involves the experts who advise the FDA on approving new medications. When a pharmaceutical company wishes to bring a new product to market, the FDA typically gathers an advisory panel to review the company's studies and advise the FDA whether to approve the drug for marketing, and under what conditions. The FDA almost always accepts the panel's recommendations. The academic doctors on these panels are supposed to have no financial ties to the company or product on which they are advising, but as the article documents, many of these "neutral" experts receive substantial research funding and lecture fees **after** the drug is approved. The investigation also found that many of the panel members had received financial support from the drug maker or key competitors for consulting, travel, lectures or research, support that was not publicly released.

Another way to increase the use of new, but not necessarily better, products is by showering doctors with coupons that reduce patients' co-pays for the new drugs. Most insurance plans that cover prescriptions have different levels of co-pays. Generic drugs may be available for no or a low co-pay, while branded drugs come with a higher co-pay, if they are covered at all. The manufacturer of a new branded drug can give out coupons that reduce the patients' co-pays, eliminating the barrier to the patient and increasing use of the new drug. The coupon system does not reduce the cost to the insurer, and in the long run does not help the patient, since most of these coupons are only available for a limited time. When the out-of-pocket cost goes up, both doctor and patient may be reluctant to switch from a medicine that seems to be working, thus repaying—many times—the subsidy initially offered. Even after generic atorvastatin became available, hundreds of thousands of patients continued to use branded Lipitor, at an estimated excess total cost of $2.1 billion between 2012 and 2014. In 2014, a study of actual out-of-pocket costs found lower costs to patients who used coupons to buy

Lipitor instead of the generic atorvastatin, while the overall cost to society rose.

Arbitrary drug expiration dates and improper packaging are another way large amounts of money are wasted. Numerous studies have shown that pills remain fully effective long after the expiration date printed on the bottle, yet millions of dollars are literally thrown away annually by hospitals and nursing homes that are obliged to do this, as well as by patients who believe what is written on the label. Injectable drugs are often sold in amounts that require unused portions to be thrown away. If a standard dose is 500 mg in 90 percent of cases, why sell it in vials of 600 mg, unless your purpose is to sell 20 percent more drug with no effort?

Another predatory practice which has come to light in recent years is paying generic manufacturers to keep a competing generic off the market. The generic company gets a handsome sum for doing nothing and the big pharmaceutical company keeps its monopoly and high prices longer. When this is not feasible, a more brute force technique is used. Brand-name drug makers realized recently that they could block generic competition by refusing to sell samples of their products to the companies who wanted to sell lower cost copies. For approval of a generic drug, the FDA requires "bioequivalence testing," using samples to show that the generics are the same as the branded product. With no branded product available for comparison, this testing could not be done. The pharmaceutical companies could do this by citing safety rules that restrict sales of certain medications with dangerous side effects. Without brand-name samples to compare, generic manufacturers cannot test their own products and prove to the FDA that they are equivalent. A classic "catch 22." In 2016, the FDA reported that it had received more than 150 inquiries from generic manufacturers that could not obtain samples for bioequivalence testing. This delay gives the brand-name companies months or years of additional freedom from generic competition.

How valid are the "safety concerns"? Let me give you one example. An old drug that has been recycled into a highly profitable "new" drug is thalidomide. This was originally sold in the 1950s and 1960s as a sedative, and was also used to treat morning sickness in pregnant women. It was taken off the market when it was found to cause severe birth defects if used by pregnant women. It has been reintroduced into medical use as a very helpful and well-tolerated treatment for multiple myeloma, a cancer of the blood and bones that has been difficult to treat. (It is also used now for the much rarer, in the United States, skin lesions caused by leprosy.) The current manufacturer of thalidomide, marketed as Thalomide, claims that it is not safe to be given out because "even a single dose can cause irreversible debilitating birth defects if not properly handled and dispensed." Well, gee whiz, matches can cause dangerous fires if they are not safely handled. Does that mean we cannot buy matches? Does Celgene Pharmaceuticals believe that the generic manufacturers are going to be giving the drug, now used to treat a disease of older adults, to pregnant women?

Recently, a clever legal maneuver has expanded the lengths to which pharmaceutical companies can go to keep generic competition at bay. In September 2017, Allergan announced that it had transferred the six patents for its blockbuster drug for dry eyes, Restasis, to the Saint Regis Mohawk Tribe, a federally recognized Indian tribe of about 15,000 members in upstate New York. The tribe received an upfront payment of $13.75 million and is eligible for up to $15 million in annual royalties, a significant amount of money for a tribe with an annual budget of $50 million. Why this generosity from Allergan? They had recently been sued by several generic manufacturers alleging that their patents were invalid because they either were not novel or were obvious in light of earlier work. The Saint Regis Mohawk Tribe, now the owner of the patents, claimed "sovereign immunity" to prevent the suits from going forward. This legal doctrine is generally used by the federal or state governments to limit suits, but also can be used by federally recognized Indian tribes. Whether this maneuver holds up in court has yet to be tested, but you have to give Allergan an A+ for shameful effort.

This blatant use of force to keep generics from cutting into their profits is not a new phenomenon. Back in 1987, Boots Pharmaceuticals, later taken over by Knoll Pharmaceuticals in New Jersey, gave a $250,000 grant to Dr. Betty Dong of the University of California, San Francisco. The purpose of the grant was to fund a study comparing the branded drug, Synthroid, against generic forms of levothyroxine. Levothyroxine is used by about eight million Americans to treat symptoms of an underactive thyroid. Both Dr. Dong and Boots were sure that the study would show the superiority of the branded product. The study ran from 1987 to 1990 and concluded that, for most patients, the generics were just as effective as the branded product. After learning these results, the sponsor refused to allow the study to be published and used threats of legal action to delay publication when Dr. Dong submitted it in 1994. After much negative publicity, the sponsor finally relented and allowed publication in 1995.

How likely is all this to change? The industry spends enormous amounts of money on campaigns and lobbyists to be sure that change is unlikely. In the 2016 election cycle, the pharmaceutical industry spent more than $58 million in campaign contributions to members of Congress and presidential candidates. In the first quarter of 2017, the pharmaceutical and health products industry spent $78 million on lobbying, far more than did any other sector of the economy. Nearly every week that Congress is in session, the industry holds fundraisers at private clubs and restaurants to help bankroll the re-election campaigns of its supporters. In 2016, Republican Representative John Shimkus of Illinois helped save billions of dollars for pharmaceutical companies by persuading the Obama administration to kill a program that was intended to lower the cost of drugs paid for under Medicare Part B. He led the effort in the House by collecting 242 signatures from members challenging the program and co-sponsoring legislation to block it. Not surprisingly, in the last election cycle, Mr. Shimkus received nearly $300,000 in contributions from the drug industry.

Not only does Big Pharma pour hundreds of millions of dollars into influencing federal policy, it does not hesitate to pour money into fighting state-level policies that might reduce its profits. PhRMA, the trade organization of the drug manufacturers, spent $64 million to help defeat a California proposal that state agencies would pay no more for drugs than does the Veterans Administration. In Louisiana, where a law was being considered that would force manufacturers to make drug prices clearer to consumers, PhRMA gave huge contributions directly to state legislators before they were to vote on the law.

A wonderful example is provided by Novo Nordisk, a major supplier of insulin, the life-saving medication that was once cheap but was now forcing my patient Jack to choose between his medication and his beloved dog. The wholesale price of a vial of Levemir, a long-acting insulin, went from $144.80 in 2012 to $335.70 in January 2017. In 2016, the soaring prices of its insulin products was causing public backlash. Investors drove down its stock price, fearing that regulators would take some action and hurt its profits. A Massachusetts law firm sued the company and two others on behalf of patients who were having trouble affording their insulin. One possible response from Novo Nordisk would have been to lower prices. Instead, the pharmaceutical giant ratcheted up its spending on lobbying. The company's political action committee spent $405,000 in 2017 on federal campaign donations, nearly double its allocation for 2015, and higher than in the election year of 2016. Novo Nordisk also spent $3.2 million in 2017 lobbying Congress and federal agencies, its highest ever spending on this activity.

To show how low the pharmaceutical companies are willing to stoop, we only have to look at the news that came out in May 2018 about how Novartis, one of the world's biggest drug makers, signed a one year, $1.2 million contract with Michael Cohen in February 2017. Mr. Cohen, President Trump's "fixer," had zero experience in pharmaceuticals or regulatory affairs, but he promised help gaining access to Trump and other officials in the new administration.

President Trump campaigned on a promise to bring down drug prices, but his long-awaited plan revealed in May 2018 largely spared the industry any real hardship, resulting in rising stock prices of the pharmaceutical industry. The Golden Rule still seems to apply: he who has the gold, rules.

Chapter 11

Enter the Middlemen

Drug prices as set by their manufacturers are bad enough, but consumer gouging happens in other ways, as well. Rarely do medications go directly from manufacturer to patients or doctors. At a minimum, you have the pharmacies that have their own add-on costs. A good pharmacist may actually earn this mark-up by checking for interactions with other medicines a patient may be taking, and by answering patient questions.

There are two other players in this drama, however, who add no value but lots of profits. First, there are now three big wholesalers in the United States, whose profits last year exceeded that of Starbucks, for adding nothing but some warehouses and trucks. Then there are the "pharmacy benefit managers," or PBMs, who ultimately decide what you are going to pay for any prescription, and who add only red tape in return for huge profits. PBMs are primarily responsible for developing and maintaining the formularies that control which medicines are covered, contracting with pharmacies, negotiating discounts and rebates with drug manufacturers, and processing and paying prescription drug claims. They work with commercial health insurers, self-insured companies and Medicare Part D programs and claim to be trying to lower prescriptions costs while maintaining quality. As of 2016, PBMs managed pharmacy benefits for 266 million Americans. There are fewer than 30 companies in this category in the US, and three major PBMs (Express Scripts, CVS Caremark, and OptumRx) comprise 68 percent of the market and cover 180 million enrollees. There have been numerous complaints about conflicts of interest, with the PBMs more interested in maximizing their profits than in lowering costs for the patients. One wonderful example is in the famous co-pay, the amount you pay after your insurance company pays its share.

When you go to pick up a prescription and are told your share, or co-pay, is $20, do you think that you are paying $20 but your insurance company is paying the rest? This may be true, but it is not uncommon for the actual cost of the drug to be $6, with the drug benefit manager taking the extra $14 as income! Under strictly enforced contracts, the pharmacist is forbidden to tell you that if you pay cash, the bottle of pills will cost you $6 rather than $20. A study published in 2018 found that approximately 28 percent of prescriptions filled for generic drugs had this wonderful little bonus for your drug insurer included. Pharmacies dare not anger the PBM by letting you in on this little secret or they may find themselves excluded from the PBM network and lose many customers.

Since the PBMs are primarily interested in maximizing their profits, they are constantly playing roulette with the drugs covered. While they portray themselves as keen negotiators who squeeze the pharmaceutical companies to get better deals that save money for patients and insurance companies, they in fact have no loyalty to either insurers or patients. They negotiate ceaselessly with drug manufacturers to get good deals, and in return promise the manufacturers preferred status and more sales. This is the usual reason why the medicine you were told you had to use to get good coverage in December becomes a high co-pay drug in January. In the meantime, the PBMs get huge rebates from the manufacturers, which are entirely hidden from public view.

Scott Gottlieb, Commissioner of the Food and Drug Administration, repeatedly has pointed out how the PBMs keep for themselves a large portion of any discounts and rebates they negotiate based on their huge buying power. It is in their interest for list prices to stay high, as their percentage also stays high! Their activities increase rather than decrease overall medication costs, as documented in a detailed investigation by *The Columbus Dispatch,* an Ohio newspaper.

They may not help your health, but the PBMs are very healthy for their shareholders. Express Scripts earns billions of dollars in profits while having less than $1 billion of physical assets and no research or development costs. They reported 2017 earnings of $5 billion on $100 billion in revenue. CVS Health includes their CVS Caremark PBM, which by itself earned $4.8 billion in 2017 on $130.6 billion in revenue.

Chapter 12

Waste

Medicine is unlike most consumer transactions. When you go to buy a car, you generally know what type and size of car you want, and usually have ample time to research different models, compare prices and haggle with the dealer. When you are sick, you tend to rely on a doctor to tell you what to do, and rarely have the time to research alternatives. While this is slowly changing in the age of the Internet, generally the medical visit is not an exchange among equals. This opens the way for doctors to provide care that is of limited value. The fact that many pointless services are "free," in that insurance covers most of the cost, makes it even less likely that patients will question the need for the suggested test(s) or treatments.

A study conducted by the National Academy of Medicine concluded that in 2016, $210 billion dollars was spent on unneeded medical care.

In a 2017 survey commissioned by the American Board of Internal Medicine (ABIM) Foundation, more than three out of four US physicians said that the frequency with which most doctors order unnecessary medical tests and procedures is a serious problem for America's health care system—and 69 percent said the average physician orders unnecessary medical tests and procedures at least once a week.

Examples abound. As younger doctors depend more and more on tests and have less and less confidence in their physical exam skills, the use of imaging has gone up. An echocardiogram is a non-invasive but expensive test that gives beautiful pictures of the working of the heart muscle and valves. During my residency training, we learned how to listen to the heart and gain much of what we needed to know about the functioning of the heart valves from the sounds. Through this process (called auscultation) we learned to distinguish the very common harmless "functional" murmur from a murmur suggesting an abnormal valve. Nowadays, the resident doctors do not feel confident that they can do this, and so order echocardiograms much more often than necessary. Many practicing doctors do the same. The chief echo technician at my hospital once lamented to me that the most common reason for physicians to order an echocardiogram was the fact that the patient had a heart!

A cardiology group to which I referred gets an ECG (electrocardiogram) on every patient at every visit even though the value of an ECG in an asymptomatic patient who has recently had one is close to zero. The national cardiology specialty society recommends against such "routine" ECGs. The patients suffer no harm from the testing, which is painless, and the individual cost is not high, but repeated hundreds of times a week, the cost mounts. Another example: a gastroenterology group I know requires all patients over 65 to have a "pre-colonoscopy visit" with their nurse practitioner to be sure they are healthy enough to have the procedure, even if they are marathon runners. A simple phone call to the primary care physician would provide the same information at no cost, but the visit fattens their bottom line. Another: the national organization of ophthalmologists has gone on record as saying patients do not need a medical evaluation before cataract surgery, as the surgery is so low-risk. At least in Massachusetts, however, no patient can have this surgery without a "medical clearance," requiring a visit to their primary care physician and usually including an ECG.

If you have ever been a hospital patient, you are doubtless familiar with the daily visit from the phlebotomist for your daily blood work. Do you need all these tests? In at least 75 percent of cases, you do not. Daily labs were ordered when you were admitted, and no one ever questioned how long they were needed or thought to cancel them as you recovered. In this case, there is the added annoyance and discomfort of a needle stick as well as the economic waste.

A study reported in *JAMA Internal Medicine* in 2018 looked at testing done in patients admitted to a hospital with cellulitis, an infection of the skin. Guidelines recommend against routinely ordering blood cultures or imaging with X-rays or ultrasound, but the tests are still widely done. They found that 30 percent of such patients had blood cultures and 70 percent had an X-ray and/or ultrasound and concluded that these "clinically useless" tests cost more than $225 million annually across the country.

Sinusitis is a common reason for doctor visits. While most cases are viral and will respond to decongestants, antibiotics are often prescribed unnecessarily. Even in those cases where there is a real need for antibiotics, guidelines suggest five to seven days of treatment, but a study published in March of 2018 found that the median duration of antibiotics was 10 days.

Much of what doctors do is out of habit, and habits die hard. Most hospital patients at one time or another get supplemental oxygen via a mask or nasal cannula. If the patient has low oxygen levels, the oxygen will make them feel better and may improve their outcome. What about the many patients receiving oxygen whose blood oxygen is normal or near-normal? Surely it does no harm, right? Wrong! Since about 2016, there has been increasing evidence that oxygen given to patients who do not need it may be harmful. A study published in the British journal *The Lancet* in 2018 looked at all the trials studying routine oxygen use and showed conclusively that those getting "liberal use" of oxygen had a 14 percent higher death rate than those who did not. Does anyone want to bet how long it will be before "routine" oxygen use is no longer routine? If I were you, I'd bet on many years hence.

Doctors order many tests because they do not have access to the results of tests you already have had. Electronic medical records were supposed to reduce this problem, but current EMRs exist in their own silos, unable to communicate with different EMRs. It is often easier and more efficient for the doctor to reorder the test than to track down the prior result. There is little incentive for this change without an external mandate, as the EMR companies want to tie the hospitals and doctors using their system to it and make changing systems difficult. Hospitals see no fiscal reason to allow outside providers to access their data, as sharing this information would make it easier for patients to leave their system. I never understood why I could go to a bank machine in almost any small town in the world and check my bank balance, yet not be able to find the results of tests my patients had performed at a hospital located 15 miles away without calling and requesting the results be faxed.

Another area where harm—as well as monetary waste—may ensue is in prescribing unnecessary medication. Giving antibiotics for viral illnesses is a rampant problem: they do not help and may do serious harm. Over the last 10 years, I cared for three elderly patients hospitalized because of the severe illness called C. diff enterocolitis. All three had high fevers, intractable diarrhea and abdominal pain. This illness, which occurs when antibiotics kill off the healthy bacteria that inhabit our gut and allow Clostridium difficile to flourish, is becoming more common. All three eventually recovered, but one had to have major surgery and was left with a colostomy. In addition to causing serious colitis, antibiotics are one of the more common causes of drug rashes and other adverse events.

As we have all become more aware of the problem of opioid abuse, doctors are looking for other ways to treat pain. There has been a rapid growth in the use of the drugs gabapentin and pregabalin to treat all kinds of pain, even though they are only approved to treat very specific kinds of pain from damaged nerves. Use of these drugs (brand named Neurontin and Lyrica) jumped 64 percent between 2012 and 2016, even though they have been found completely ineffective for conditions such as chronic back pain, for which they are widely prescribed. Again, this is not only a waste of money, but the drugs have many serious side effects including dizziness, fatigue and visual disturbance.

In 2012, the American Board of Internal Medicine began a program called "Choosing Wisely," which **appeared** to be a worthwhile effort. The Board asked specialty societies to suggest five tests or procedures used in their specialty that were of little value and whose use should be questioned. When first released in April, 2012, nine specialty societies contributed information; now there are more than 500 recommendations from 80 specialty societies. On the surface, this seemed like a great idea: ask the experts who order them which tests and procedures are over-used or performed unnecessarily. However, skeptics, including myself, note that in most cases these recommendations do not target the tests and procedures that bring in high income to the specialists, but instead target those that are rarely done and/or are not very lucrative to practitioners in that specialty. For example, the American Academy of Orthopedic Surgeons submitted the following five recommendations:

A) Avoid routine post-operative ultrasound looking for phlebitis after elective hip or knee replacement. (Test done by hospital; no revenue to orthopedist.)

B) Don't use needle lavage (i.e. washing out with sterile water) for symptomatic osteoarthritis of the knee. (A poorly-paid procedure for which much higher paid alternatives abound.)

C) Don't use glucosamine/chondroitin pills for symptomatic osteoarthritis of the knee. (Again, loss of revenue to the pharmacy, not the orthopedist.)

D) Don't use wedge insoles for symptomatic osteoarthritis of the knee. (Ditto.)

E) Don't use post-operative splinting of the wrist after carpal tunnel release surgery. (Ditto.)

What all these recommendations have in common is that avoiding them will have zero impact on the income of the specialists who made the recommendations. Conspicuously absent is reference to a procedure such as partial menisectomy (removal of cartilage) for patients with knee pain and nontraumatic partial tears of the meniscus. This procedure has been shown to have no benefit compared to simple observation without surgery (see: Annals of the Rheumatic Diseases February 2018), but it **is** a highly lucrative procedure for the orthopedic surgeons who do the surgeries.

While I have picked orthopedic surgery for this example, I could do the same for most of the suggestions made by other specialties. They were all very careful to make suggestions that were sensible, harmless and did not impact their members' incomes.

Americans undergo more high-cost surgical procedures— including hip and knee replacements and cardiac stenting—than do Canadians or most Europeans. While this may in some cases be a good thing—it is easier for an elderly person to get joint replacement surgery, which may improve their quality of life, in the US than in Canada—it often represents over-expectation about the results expected. The joint replacement pre-op process focuses entirely on the details of the process, and virtually never on what is to be expected as a long-term outcome or what alternatives are available. It has been shown repeatedly that when proper teaching is done, with a balanced presentation about what results to expect and what the patient will experience, fewer people opt for surgery.

Prostate cancer is the third most common cancer in men and is often over-treated. Patients with lower grades of prostate cancer have a cancer-related mortality of only 2.4 percent after 10 years of watching with no treatment (and this is a cancer that typically hits elderly men). Treatment has many side-effects, including loss of bladder control, impotence and bowel issues. Despite this, most men with low-risk prostate cancer choose surgery or radiation over observation. The treatment they choose seems to depend mostly on whom they see. For a typical low-risk patient, 93 percent of urologic surgeons recommend surgery and 72 percent of radiation oncologists recommend radiation! Rarely do men make truly informed decisions. In a survey of men with newly diagnosed prostate cancer, more than half greatly overestimated the survival benefit of the proposed treatment, and more than half of those who had already seen a urologist got most of the questions wrong on a test designed to see if they understood their disease.

Coronary disease is a common problem, and treatment can include some combination of lifestyle changes, medications, stenting and surgery. Putting a stent into a closed artery that has caused an acute heart attack definitely and substantially benefits patients. Stents also help reduce symptoms in patients who have angina pectoris (chest pain that comes with increased physical activity) that is interfering with their life. Many patients have milder, stable angina. It has been shown that for patients with stable angina pectoris, stenting offers no benefit over optimal medical therapy in terms of either long-term survival or quality of life, but this procedure is still often recommended. It is an easy sell by the cardiologist. "See, you have this partially blocked artery. I can fix this by opening it up and putting in a stent." Who would want to walk around with a blocked artery? Rarely is the patient told that the procedure will not make them live any longer or see a major change in their daily life, or that having the stent means they will have to take blood thinners that may produce serious bleeding problems. They are told they have a blockage that should be fixed.

Useless surgeries abound in orthopedics. Take spinal fusion, an operation that welds together vertebrae to try to relieve pain from worn-out disks. There were four trials done in the early 2000s that showed surgery was no better than physical therapy in relieving back pain. Despite this convincing evidence that the surgery was useless, spinal fusion surgery was used **more** often in the United States after these trials were published. Only after many Blue Cross plans refused to pay for it did rates decline.

A procedure called vertebroplasty, used to help back pain due to a collapsed vertebra, involves injecting material into a collapsed vertebra to expand it. In 2009, two trials were published in the prestigious *New England Journal of Medicine* from two different groups, both showing the procedure was no better than a sham operation. The same thing was shown again in a more recent trial, published in the New England Journal in June 2018. (A sham operation is one in which the patient is sedated, has a needle placed or superficial cut made and sewn up, and is told he had the procedure being studied, even though nothing was really done.) Despite this, the procedure is still widely used. Many back surgeries are not only useless but make patients worse. Look at Tiger Woods, who has had four surgeries and is still struggling. Look at basketball coach Steve Kerr who missed the majority of the 2016-17 season because of complications from back surgery.

Doctors continue to inject hyaluronic acid into arthritic knees, despite ample evidence that this is useless and that guidelines from the American Academy of Orthopedic Surgeons, published in 2013, gave a strong recommendation against doing this.

There are several reasons why doctors continue to perform clinically useless procedures. New drugs must be subjected to clinical trials and show their safety and efficacy before the FDA lets them on the market, but there is no such requirement for surgical procedures. There is a huge placebo effect for procedures, and many doctors are impressed that their patients seem to do better after an operation, never considering that the patient may have done just as well with acupuncture, chiropractic or a sham operation. While I hate to say so, there is also the huge financial incentive for the doctor to "do something," even if doing so has little or no benefit for the patient.

Chapter 13

Fraud

While I was in active practice, at least several times every week I would get a fax asking me to "sign the attached document" so that my patient could get diabetic supplies, a motorized scooter or an electric lift chair. I would ask my secretary to call the patient to confirm the request, and nine times out of 10 he or she had not requested the supplies or equipment. In most of the remaining 10 percent, the patients had been contacted by phone and told they could get the equipment at no cost if their doctor approved it. These scams are rampant, and if even a small percentage of doctors sign these forms, hundreds of millions of dollars are charged to Medicare for unneeded supplies.

In 2017, the New York King County District Attorney indicted 20 individuals (including four doctors) and 14 corporations for a massive fraud operation that had cheated Medicare and Medicaid out of approximately $146 million over three years. The scheme involved recruiters going into low-income areas and offering cash payments to individuals who had a Medicare or Medicaid card and were willing to be transported to a clinic, where they were put through a wide variety of medically unnecessary tests. This is hardly an isolated example. The payoff for such schemes is so potentially lucrative that similar schemes are widespread, and if the perpetrators are smart enough to get out before they are caught, they can cost the health care system billions of dollars every year.

In March of 2018, a Pennsylvania hospital and cardiology group paid $20 million to resolve "kickback" allegations. The suit alleged that between 1999 and 2010, the hospital paid a local cardiology group up to $2 million a year to refer patients to the hospital for services that were either duplicative or not even performed. The way this came to light was through a suit brought by a "whistle blower," a doctor formerly employed by the group. Similar stories abound. Mercy Health, a 23-hospital group based in Cincinnati paid $14 million to resolve allegations that they paid an oncologist and five internists to refer patients to their hospitals. In Massachusetts, a urologist has filed a whistle-blower suit against Steward Healthcare, alleging that he was strongly pressured to refer patients only to Steward hospitals even when he felt they would receive better care at a different facility. He claimed that when he resisted and referred patients elsewhere, his patients would be called at home by Steward representatives and told their appointments had to be changed.

A subtler form of fraud lies in the Medicare Advantage plans, a congressionally-mandated program that allows seniors to enroll in a type of HMO for their care. These plans receive a fixed annual fee per member, per year, to provide all their medical care. In 2017, about 19 million of the 56 million Medicare enrollees chose one of these plans. The amounts paid are adjusted based on the health status of the enrollees, to protect the plans from having unusual numbers of very sick, high-cost enrollees, Not surprisingly, the plans are tempted to make their enrollees seem sicker than they are to drive up the amounts they receive. A congressional auditor testified in July of 2017 that more than $16 billion in extra payments were improperly paid to these plans in 2016 because of inflated estimates of how sick their enrollees were.

Similarly, as reported in *The Wall Street Journal* in March of 2018, major health insurers use a technique known as "cross-walking" to boost their revenues by millions of dollars. This involves merging a patient's original health plan with one ranked higher by Medicare (which uses a five-star scale) that gives bonuses to providers for higher quality. The shift boosts a plan's rating without requiring any actual improvement in quality. For Humana, the shift was estimated to have increased their revenues by nearly $600 million in 2018.

Another grey area lies in how the discharge diagnosis is assigned. Since hospitals are paid a lump sum by Medicare based on the patient's final diagnosis, there is great pressure on attending physicians to pick a diagnosis that generates a higher payment. Many times, having discharged a patient with a diagnosis of pneumonia or urinary tract infection, a medical records clerk would approach me to ask if I would consider changing the diagnosis to Sepsis, a disease with a higher charge. I usually said no, but I was not beholden to the hospital. Now that most inpatient care is under "hospitalists," I wonder how much more often the upcoding will be done. These physicians have no independent practice and know they can be replaced if they are labelled uncooperative.

The electronic medical record has had minimal effect on improving the quality of patient care, but it has helped doctors "upcode" to generate a higher payment for a visit. When a few clicks of the mouse allow the doctor to add reams of normal findings to a note, it is very easy to make a short visit look like a comprehensive visit, with a higher reimbursement. I sent "Tony" (again, not his real name) to a neurosurgeon for an opinion about his ongoing sciatica. I can vividly recall seeing the surgeon's note describing a very detailed medical history—covering his prior health, allergies, and medications used—as well as a head-to-toe physical exam, including retinal exam and examination of the genitals and rectum! When I saw Tony in my office and asked him what Dr. X had done, Tony said, "He tapped on my reflexes and reviewed the CAT scan with me."

This "cut and paste" school of note generation, in which the history and physical from prior visits is brought forward and every lab and X-ray report is pasted into the note, is a pervasive problem. With this creative writing exercise, a visit lasting 10 minutes may be accompanied by a 10-page note! This note is then used to justify a higher level of service than was provided. It would be simply annoying to the referring doctor and a bit more expensive to the insurance company if the only effect was a higher billing charge, but this style of "note inflation" is often dangerous, because it becomes very difficult for the referring physician reading this massive tome to figure out what was actually done at the most recent visit. Emergency departments use specific billing codes to indicate the severity of the illness. Between 2006 and 2010, hospital claims for the top two levels increased from 40 percent to 54 percent of submitted bills. It seems very unlikely that patients suddenly got much sicker. Much more likely is that upcoding became more pervasive when a few mouse clicks could generate a much more detailed note.

I did not know whether to include this next topic under Fraud or Lawyers, as it involves lawyers encouraging fraud! *The New York Times* in April ran a story describing how women who had undergone surgery for pelvic organ prolapse that included use of mesh implants were targeted for the benefit of law firms. There is a huge class action lawsuit underway against the manufacturers of mesh implants, but the lawyers found that settlements were much higher for the women who had the implants surgically removed than for those whose implants remained in place. Well, an obvious way to juice up the payments and their fees was to convince more women to have the mesh removed! Women were cold-called by marketers and convinced that their lives were at stake, and that they could have the implants removed at no cost. They were flown to Florida or Georgia, where they had the surgery at outpatient centers, and flown home. In the cases described in the New York Times article, many of these women who had had few or no symptoms before the surgical removal were left much worse, often unable to control their bladder. Also, the women's upfront costs, including the surgery, were paid for by finance firms at very high interest rates, to be paid from the expected settlements. Between finance charges and legal fees, very little of the settlements ever reached the affected women.

As new and exciting scientific advances are trumpeted in the news media, our expectations of medical miracles increase, and new areas of fraud open up via non-existent breakthroughs. A recent example is Theranos, a start-up that claimed to have developed a portable analyzer that could perform virtually any medical test using only a drop of blood. Despite the lack of any independent studies of their technology, defended as necessary to protect their trade secrets, the public was sold on Theranos and their stock price soared. Now that we know it was all a sham, a "Potemkin village" show, we are left to wonder how many other "breakthroughs" are real. (A Potemkin village is an impressive facade or show designed to hide an undesirable fact or condition. It is named after an eighteenth century Russian politician, Grigori Potemkin, who supposedly built facades of prosperous villages along a route that Catherine the Great was to travel to fool her into believing the area was more prosperous that it was.)

I cannot end a chapter on fraud without discussing the internet. In the winter of 2017-18, the website *YourNewsWire* published a story with the headline "CDC Doctor: 'Disastrous' Flu Shot is Causing Deadly Flu Outbreak." The story quoted an anonymous physician, who supposedly worked at the Centers for Disease Control and Prevention, warning that nearly everyone dying of the flu had gotten flu shots. He was quoted as saying, "This scares the crap out of me." This story rapidly spread, getting about 500,000 shares on Facebook in January alone and generating thousands of online comments. The problem was that this story was fabricated: no such physician existed. I can only cringe at the thought of how many people avoided getting flu shots because of this story. "Fake Medical News" has become big business. There are hundreds of websites purveying fake news, for a variety of purposes. The most obvious is to sell products of dubious value and bilk consumers. Websites also can garner many "clicks" and turn these into advertising dollars. While fake medical news is hardly a new phenomenon—think of the magic elixirs that were peddled out of wagons in the nineteenth century—it has become a much larger problem in the internet age. The decline of traditional print media, with editors and fact-checkers, has led to a proliferation of credible-sounding but totally erroneous information. For example, only about half of people prescribed a cholesterol-lowering drug are still taking it after six months. While there is debate among doctors as to whether people with no heart disease should take these drugs, there is unanimity that those with coronary disease live longer and have fewer recurrent heart attacks if the drugs are used. Despite this, if you type "statin risks" into a search engine, you get over 3.5 million "hits." Is it any wonder that patients who do not have a trusting relationship with their doctor decide to stop this "dangerous" drug on their own?

While the Federal Trade Commission has the authority to crack down on fraudulent advertising, the same websites just pop up under new names.

Chapter 14

## How Do We Want to End Our Days?

Some years earlier, the hospital to which I admitted patients switched to a "hospitalist" model. Teams of mostly young, right-out-of-residency doctors took over the care of patients in the hospital, sending them back to their primary care physicians after discharge. The hospital executives liked this because having doctors there all the time meant that if patients could be discharged at 6 pm, they would be, instead of waiting until their attending primary care doctor rounded the following morning. Length of stay could be reduced and the hospital's bottom line improved. Many primary care doctors liked the switch as well, because coming to the hospital to see one or two patients was not as efficient a use of their time as staying in their offices. While I have to admit this system probably extended my career a few years—no more exhausting 2 am phone calls about a patient who had taken a turn for the worse—I still felt that continuity of care was lost and that patient outcomes were not as good. My compromise was to go to the hospital a couple of days a week when my patients were admitted to both reassure them that I had not forgotten them and to intercede when I felt their care was suboptimal.

One morning I went to the Intensive Care Unit to see "Harry" (not his real name), an 82-year-old retired fire fighter, father of six and grandfather of 23. Harry had late-stage congestive heart failure due to a weakened heart muscle. He had been in and out of the hospital seven times in the preceding two years. If he were younger, he would have been listed for a heart transplant, but he was too old for this to be an option under national guidelines. Instead, he would come to the emergency department, increasingly short of breath, and be admitted. His medicines would be increased or adjusted and he would get better briefly. The intervals between his admissions were getting shorter. On this admission, he had already been in the ICU for eight days, and the medicine designed to help his breathing was making his kidneys worse. When I went into his room, Harry was sitting bolt upright, laboring to breath, with two IV lines and oxygen mask in place, and a catheter in his bladder. His first words were: "Doc, please get them to let me go home. You and I know this is not doing any good and I just want to be home."

The old saying has it that nothing is sure but death and taxes. If you have good lawyers and accountants, you may be able to figure out a way to avoid taxes, but the other half remains true. Even with all the money in the world and the best medical care available, none of us is here forever. The oldest person alive in the United States is 113, and the oldest person ever documented died at 122. The job of the medical profession is to try to see that each of us lives out our allotted lifespan as well as possible, and that none of us dies of preventable or treatable conditions. A huge dilemma for patients, families and doctors is to know when death is inevitable and when treatment is more meddlesome than helpful.

End-of-life care represents a major challenge because it is often of little benefit to the patients, affects many people and is very expensive. Many patients dying in the United States receive medical care that gives little or no improvement in their outcome and is all-too-often at odds with their wishes. Even though 80 percent of patients say that hospitalization or ICU stays at the end of life impose unwanted burdens, about one third of deaths in this country occur in the hospital. It has been estimated that 25 percent of Medicare payments go to patients in their last year of life. The key question is not cost, but value: are we spending hundreds of billions of dollars on care that does not help patients but may instead harm them?

In pulp novels and Western movies, "die like a dog" is intended to describe a horrible death, but in contemporary American society, dogs are often allowed to die much more comfortably and peacefully than humans. Most pet owners have had the sad experience of realizing that their beloved companion is suffering, and they allow their veterinarian to euthanize the cat or dog. We went through this with our own aged cats, and though we cried, we knew the decision was what was best for the animal. We do not, however, usually allow our sick, aged relatives to die peacefully on their own.

Let me be clear that I am not simply talking about chronologic age. Unlike Ezekiel Emanuel, I do NOT want to die at 75, nor, I suspect, will he when he gets closer. (Emanuel penned the infamous article in *The Atlantic Monthly* laying out the case that by 75 he would have lived a full life and did not want to live with increasing frailty and be a burden to his family or society.) I have had numerous patients who lived healthy active lives well into their eighties. What I **am** talking about is futility. Generally, doctors are fairly accurate in their assessment about how likely a sick hospitalized patient is to survive, but they seem reluctant to share this information with the patients and their families. All too often I have heard the hospital staff talk about doing this and doing that, when they knew, all too well, that neither this nor that would do anything but extend life by a few days at the cost of much pain and suffering.

A very large portion of health care spending occurs during the last weeks and months of a person's life—usually because of hospital, and particularly intensive care unit, stays. About a quarter of all Medicare recipients die in the hospital. Some of this is unavoidable. A patient may be admitted for a planned surgery and suffer a complication, or an infection that would normally respond to treatment and lead to recovery may turn out to be resistant to antibiotics. In this case, the hospital admission and associated costs are unfortunate but appropriate. In all too many situations, however, the (usually elderly) patient has severe end-stage disease, and the doctors caring for them know that death is inevitable and soon. In this situation, are we caring for them by admitting them to an ICU and postponing the inevitable death by a few days or weeks, at the cost of great discomfort and dehumanization? When asked, most elders would prefer to die at home, in comfort and surrounded by their loved ones and not surrounded by strangers in the alien environment of the ICU, with tubes in every part of their body and daily, multiple blood draws in their worn-out veins.

Why the discordance between what patients say they want and the care usually provided? Part of the blame lies with doctors who are reluctant to be open and honest with their patients with a poor prognosis. It is much easier for doctors to say, "Let's try this," than to admit that no available treatment will make a major difference. It has been shown that physicians' beliefs and training influence care much more than patients' beliefs—exactly the opposite of what should happen. Part of the blame lies with families who are reluctant to accept inevitable death and insist that doctors "do everything" even when they are told it will not help. It is easy and natural to reject what the doctors are saying. "Most people like this will die soon, but not my Dad." All too often I have been in the situation where a patient has told me they are ready to accept a comfortable death, but then a child flies in from far away and insists that I "do everything." Even when there are several children who agree to let a parent die peacefully, doctors tend to heed the children who insist on aggressive care, as they are the ones who threaten to sue if their parent is not given "everything."

Focusing on treating a patient's symptoms near the end of life rather than on extending life often carries an unexpected bonus: a longer as well as a better life. There is now evidence that patients with cancer and severe heart failure live longer when enrolled in hospice and other palliative care programs. The patients with advanced heart failure who were enrolled in hospice had fewer ED visits, fewer hospital days, were less likely to die in the hospital and lived slightly longer than those getting traditional "active" care.

In 2018 we witnessed the death of Barbara Bush at 92 years of age, at home with comfort care and palliative measures. She had been diagnosed with chronic lung disease and heart failure for many years, and in the preceding year, she had been hospitalized multiple times. Given her history, age, and limited outlook for meaningful recovery, it was clear that she was likely to face recurrent hospitalizations and inevitable death despite all that medical science could offer. In the end, she decided with her family to die with quality of life, not quantity of life. She was cared for at home and her treatment focused on relieving symptoms. In her last days of life, she was enjoying the company of her husband, children and grandchildren, as well as sharing stories, drinking bourbon, and providing advice as she often did. She died peacefully on April 17, 2018, in the presence of her extended family and beloved husband.

Her death reminds us of the importance of caring for the complete patient, understanding patient and family needs, and placing quality of life as a priority over quantity of life in this type of situation. In patients with cancer or end-stage heart or lung disease, an enormous amount of resources and dollars are spent in the last six months to provide care that may not improve long-term outcomes or quality of life, and instead only extend the patients' suffering.

What about Harry? Five of Harry's six children came to accept that he was near the end and wanted to respect his wishes, but his oldest son, who lived on the west coast, insisted that the doctors keep trying to improve his heart. Eventually he acceded, and Harry got his wish. Harry went home with hospice care and died peacefully in his sleep, with children and grandchildren with him at all times.

Chapter 15

Misdiagnosis Costs and Kills

About 20 years ago, former patients who had moved to Maine called and asked if I would see their daughter who had been unable to conceive despite many doctor's visits and increasingly difficult fertility treatments. I warned them that I was hardly an expert on infertility but would be happy to see her. "Karen" (not her real name) described eight years of being unable to get pregnant. She had undergone numerous blood tests, done her basal body temperature chart so often that she hated the sight of a thermometer, and even tried IVF (in vitro fertility). Much of the care was not covered by her health insurance, and she and her husband had spent thousands of dollars trying for a baby. All her care had been managed by the doctors in the obstetrics/gynecology group in her home town.

As an otherwise apparently healthy young woman, she had no family doctor or Internist. Other than her infertility issue, she said she felt tired and did not like the cold Maine weather. Her skin was dry, her pulse slow and she had an obvious goiter (enlarged thyroid). It did not require Dr. House to immediately suspect she might have an underactive thyroid. Lab testing confirmed my suspicion. I started her on thyroid supplementation and advised her to have further testing done back home, which should be faxed to me so I could adjust the dose. Six months later I got a joyous phone call. Not only did Karen feel more energetic, she was now three months pregnant!

Diagnostic error, defined as a missed or delayed diagnosis, and/or failure to communicate that diagnosis to the patient, is a huge and widely under-appreciated problem worldwide. A report from the National Academy of Medicine entitled "Improving Diagnosis in Health Care" was released in September 2015 and brought the issue to public attention. Until that point, most patient safety initiatives had focused on the obvious errors: wrong-site surgery, giving patients medicines to which they were allergic, leaving instruments inside the body, etc. While these are clearly a problem, malpractice insurance carriers have identified failure to diagnose as the leading cause of malpractice lawsuits. Postmortem examinations over many years have consistently shown that diagnostic errors contribute to 10 percent of patient deaths.

There are many causes of diagnostic error. The patient may withhold crucial information. The doctor may fail to ask the right questions or miss something on the physical exam. Tests that doctors order may not be done, or the test results may never reach the doctor. X-rays may be misinterpreted by the radiologist. The commonest cause of missed diagnoses, however, is the one that caused so much misery to Karen and her husband: the doctor just never thought of it. Once the diagnosis was considered, it was an easy matter to both confirm and treat.

The National Academy report estimated that every American would in their lifetime be affected by a missed diagnosis, either of themselves or a family member. They stated that five percent of adults seeking outpatient care each year experience a diagnostic error. Many of these errors do not result in serious harm, but many do. Diagnostic error contributes to one in 10 patient deaths, and roughly 40-80,000 deaths each year in hospitals are linked to inaccurate or delayed diagnoses. My mother died largely because her doctors failed to consider why she was feeling so poorly after her surgery and had no appetite, but she kept faithfully taking her diabetic medication. She was suffering from a build-up of acid in her system, made much worse by the diabetic medication. When she complained, she was told to take some sherry to stimulate her appetite! By the time the real problem was discovered she had slipped into a coma from which she never recovered.

Our son had a cough and was sent for a chest X-ray, which was reported as normal. When his cough persisted, I asked a pulmonary specialist—who was thorough enough to ask him to bring the X-ray to the visit—to see him. After an examination and a review of the X-ray, he said: "I have good news and bad news. The good news is that your cough is due to postnasal drip and can be helped with some over-the-counter medicine. The bad news is that your X-ray is NOT normal." Our son, in fact, had enlarged lymph nodes that were subsequently diagnosed as being due to Hodgkin's disease. He has done well, but we will never know whether he might have been able to receive a less difficult course of treatment had the board-certified radiologist not misread the "simple" chest X-ray, allowing the diagnosis to be made earlier.

Misdiagnosis has both health and financial implications. The effect on a patient's health is obvious, but the financial consequences are also real. Delayed diagnoses mean more unnecessary tests and visits, and lost wages from missed work. If you are diagnosed with a serious condition that you do not have, which happens more often than you might believe, you may miss work and be subjected to treatment that you never needed, as well as major side effects. Hospital stays are prolonged when the doctors are pursuing the wrong treatment due to a wrong diagnosis. When the Mayo Clinic did a trial using decision support to help their residents make better diagnoses, patients got out of the hospital a day earlier and at a savings of more than $1,000 per admission. Promptly making the right diagnosis is good both for the patient's health and for the bottom line.

Many tools are available to help doctors and patients arrive at the right diagnosis promptly. There are published checklists and advice for patients on how to prepare for a medical visit. I was one of the original developers and have spent more than 20 years working to improve a computer-based expert system called DXplain that accepts clinical findings (history, physical exam findings, lab test results and imaging findings) and gives the doctor a list of diseases suggested by these findings, in order of likelihood. Other systems, such as Isabel and VisualDx, are also available. We and others have shown that these systems result in better diagnostic performance by doctors who use them. The biggest impediment to the more widespread use of decision support is that doctors do not realize they need help! A fascinating study was reported in 2013 in *JAMA Internal Medicine*. The authors recruited general internists from an online community and asked them to diagnose hypothetical patients from case summaries posted online. They had both easier and more challenging cases to consider. The 118 physicians who participated correctly diagnosed 55 percent of the easier cases but only six percent of the challenging cases. What was chilling in the study findings was the degree of confidence that they were correct: 7.2 out of 10 on the easy cases, and 6.4 out of 10 on the challenging ones! I may be wrong, but I am pretty sure I am right!

Since diagnostic errors are not usually as flagrant as removing the wrong organ, many misdiagnoses are not appreciated. Only when the use of diagnostic decision support systems becomes mandatory or can be done automatically will their full potential be reached.

A "low tech" way to prevent diagnostic errors is vastly underused: a second opinion. My wife and I were playing bridge when I was asked to examine one of our fellow players, who was afraid he was having a stroke. "Mark" was complaining of weakness and tingling in both his hands. I did a brief exam and reassured him that he was not having a stroke and that if he rested for a bit and had some juice he would feel better, which he did. I also urged him to see his doctor as soon as possible for further evaluation. A few days later he called me to say that his doctor told him that he had suffered a TIA (transient ischemic attack), or temporary stroke, and wanted to put him on blood thinners. I said this seemed unlikely. (I had the advantage of seeing Mark while he was having his symptoms, while his doctor saw him when he felt fine and was recalling his symptoms.) I urged him to see a neurologist before doing anything, which he did. The neurologist agreed that this had not been a TIA and was probably related to his known migraine headaches. The neurologist reassured him that he did not need more testing or blood thinners. Doctors at the Mayo Clinic published a study showing that when patients initiated a second opinion, anywhere from 10 percent to 62 percent of those second opinions resulted in a major change in the diagnosis, treatment or prognosis.

Chapter 16

## The Electronic Record: Friend or Foe?

I once handed a prescription to a patient who looked at it and smilingly said, "You can't be a real doctor. I can read this." It is true that doctors have been notorious for poor penmanship, and I have had after-hours calls from pharmacists who could not read a prescription written by a colleague for whom I was covering. (Usually the best I could do was tell them to call in the morning to talk to the prescriber.) I also vividly recall the problems I had when doing weekend rounds in the days before hospitalists, when five of us shared night and weekend call. One of the five had such bad handwriting that he might as well have written his "sign-out" notes in Sanskrit. A typical note might be intended to convey a message such as "Mrs. Jones was admitted last Tuesday for pneumonia. She seemed much better today but still had a fever. If her fever stays away for 24 hours, you can discharge her." Dr. F's note could be read roughly as, "Mx Jxx...xxxTu...fev...24...her." After trying unsuccessfully to get him to print, I finally resorted to deciphering the room number (even that was not always easy) and asking the nurses and the patient what was needed.

Accurate and readily available information is critically important for good patient care. In addition to poor legibility, the traditional hand-written medical record had many other deficiencies. Paper charts could not always be found when needed. A chart might be needed at several places simultaneously when multiple specialists were involved in the patient's care. The sickest patients often had a record consisting of many thick volumes, and finding a specific piece of information was challenging. Laboratory test results and X-ray reports often were not put into the charts promptly, and sometimes were filed incorrectly.

The electronic record was supposed to fix all this. Expectations were so high that under the American Recovery and Reinvestment Act of 2009, the federal government poured what would eventually total more than $35 billion into incentives to get hospitals and doctors to adopt Electronic Medical Records (EMRs). The incentives worked. Over the past decade, the use of EMRs has increased dramatically. In 2008, fewer than one in 10 US hospitals had an EMR. In 2018, fewer than one in 10 do not. The increased EMR use in physicians' offices has been similar. The vision was a scenario in which all a patient's information would be available wherever they were treated, and in which computerized alerts would prevent errors and enhance care.

What we have seen, unfortunately, is a proliferation of EMRs that mimic the old paper chart in form and which exist primarily to enhance billing and assure compliance with bureaucratic demands for "quality indicators." Notes have become much longer but not more useful. All too often I hear complaints that "the doctor never looked at me. He/she spent all the time looking at the computer." This lack of eye contact is not simply an annoyance and discourtesy (though it is that!), it has measurable deleterious effects on care. Many older patients have reduced hearing and depend to some extent on lip-reading to follow what the doctor is saying, which is impossible to do when the doctor is not looking at them. Moreover, seeing how a patient replies to a question is often as important as what they are saying. An experienced clinician will pick up on clues from the patient's manner when they reply, and know when a simple yes or no needs follow-up probing and clarification. This cannot be done when the doctor is absorbed in the computer screen.

During my years as a resident and later as a teacher in the hospital, hospital "rounding" meant going as a group to the patients' bedsides and presenting their problems to the senior attending doctor. The attending could ask questions and examine the patient, perhaps pointing out physical findings the house staff had missed. The patient could in turn bring up issues that had not been addressed. Today, "rounds" all too often mean that the team gathers in a conference room and discusses "virtual patients," reviewing labs and X-ray reports and carrying on with previous erroneous information perpetuated from prior notes. Multiple studies have shown that house staff spend at least twice as much time at a computer terminal as they do with the patients.

The various EMRs almost never communicate with each other if they are not part of the same hospital system. While I can exchange emails and send Word documents to anyone in the world, all-too-often I had to depend on the fax machine to get information about a patient seen elsewhere, even if the visit was only 10 miles away. This does not only mean that I cannot interrogate an EMR from across the country; all too often I cannot interrogate an EMR in the same city.

Even legibility is still not perfect, albeit in a new manner. Many medical notes are dictated using voice recognition software, which results in many errors. A careful study comparing this form of note generation with notes transcribed by a trained medical secretary found an error rate of 7.4 out of every 100 words. Some are simply comical, such as the patient being described as both he and she in the same paragraph, but others are more substantive. Ideally, the doctor would proof every note before it is finished, but this is rarely done. Virtually every such note I received from consultants finished with a statement such as, "Generated using voice recognition software. Please excuse any typographical errors." I could pick up the he/she issue without any problem, but I was always left wondering what less obvious errors were in the note.

The EMR **should** do well at catching potential medication errors such as trying to prescribe a medication to which the patient has a listed allergy, or at picking up potential interactions of a newly-prescribed medicine with medicines the patient is currently taking. Unfortunately, a common problem with these functions is the same as the problem of alarms in the ICU. There are so many alarms, and so many are false, that the nurses in the ICU or the doctors at their EMRs tune them out and assume that since the last 10 were false alarms, the current one is as well. A news story in June 2018 described just such an event. A patient at the Good Samaritan Hospital in Brockton was given a drug to which he was severely allergic, despite this being noted in the record, and despite the fact that both the pharmacist dispensing the drug and the nurse administering it got "pop-ups" noting the allergy. Fortunately, the patient recovered, but only after being rushed to the ICU. When you see a warning pop up on your computer screen dozens or even hundreds of times a day, after a while it is easy to tune these out as more false alarms.

EMRs as currently used in most hospitals and doctors' offices unfortunately do one thing well: they contribute heavily to physician "burn-out." Physicians more and more feel like highly-paid clerical employees as they try to satisfy the demands of the EMR for endless amounts of often clinically useless data entry. Hospital-based physicians, who go to multiple workstations during their work day, must constantly sign in and out and go through password checks. An audit of one EMR showed that physicians spend almost as much time on security tasks as they do reviewing patient data. The typical 10-hour emergency department shift requires 4,000 clicks.

A 2018 Mayo Clinic study found that the leading cause of physicians' dissatisfaction with their profession is the number of hours of data entry and box-checking they must complete. A simple office visit note now often consists of four to five pages of verbiage and "mandated" information that is of little clinical value. A survey of more than 15,000 physicians by Medscape in 2018 found that 42 percent reported significant burn-out. Should you, the patient, care about physician burn-out? Yes, you should, for there is ample data showing that doctors who were on the verge of quitting the profession or had other signs of burnout made significantly more errors than their peers.

Since the major raison d'être of current EMRs is billing and compliance, not improved care, many functions that would improve care have not been implemented. I have worked on a diagnostic decision support system that has been shown to help doctors make better differential diagnoses, as have others, but since this will not improve revenue, it has been difficult to get it integrated into the EMR. The problem is not the adoption of EMRs, but rather the failure to produce one that guides doctors in their daily work and enhances their memory. The idea of using electronic records to improve care is not a new one. Some 50 years ago, Dr. Larry Weed proposed the adoption of "medical records that guide and teach," recognizing that the human memory was both finite and fallible. When he proposed this, the technology to support his ideas was not capable of implementing them. The technology we now have would allow the record to truly improve clinical care, but implementation still lags. Doctors know what they want and need to get from their electronic records, but their needs usually seem to take second place to administrative and billing needs. In large group practices or hospitals, the selection of an EMR is done by the administrators not the clinicians, and the clinicians are then forced to live with the choice.

In many instances, doctors and nurses have developed elaborate "work-arounds" to get past the barriers placed by their EMR. Hospital nurses are not supposed to give any medication that is not entered electronically, but they may ignore this rule and give a medicine based on notes they took discussing the patient with a doctor. In one hospital, the computers that the nurses rolled around the floor would malfunction periodically when in Wi-Fi dead zones, so the nurses took to using paper notes or white boards. Many doctors at the Massachusetts General Hospital are using doctors in India as "scribes" to write notes based on audio recordings made during the visit so that the doctor is more able to concentrate on the patient. As you can imagine, this is very costly, and the cost ultimately falls back on us as health consumers.

Chapter 17

## All of Us Play a Role

Pills are not the answer for an unhealthy lifestyle.

The health care system is only one factor that determines a nation's health, and not even the most important one when it comes to the health of populations. Differences in lifestyle, eating habits, exercise and culture all play a role. A widely publicized study that came out in the journal *Circulation* in April 2018 found that five healthy behaviors could add 12-14 years to the lifespan of middle-aged adults: a healthy diet, regular exercise, not smoking, maintaining a healthy weight and moderate alcohol consumption. These factors were associated with reduced rates of cancer, cardiovascular disease and overall mortality. The researchers estimated that the average life expectancy at age 50 was 14 years longer for women with all five factors compared to women with none. Among men, the added life expectancy was 12 years. If a drug or surgical procedure could come close to these benefits, its developer would be bound for Stockholm!

Even patients with diabetes, who have a much higher death rate than non-diabetics, benefit dramatically from adhering to healthy habits. Those with three or four healthy habits had less than half the rates of coronary events, strokes and deaths than those with none of these habits. (The habits studied were high-quality diet, nonsmoking, moderate-vigorous exercise and drinking alcohol in moderation.)

A huge percentage of health care spending goes to the management of chronic diseases such as diabetes, hypertension, coronary disease and chronic lung disease. Many of these diseases can be prevented with healthier lifestyles.

As a nation, the US is grossly overweight. You do not need statistics—just look around you. The statistics, however, are there. A study published in the journal *Pediatrics* in February 2018 looked at data from the National Health and Nutrition Examination Survey and found that in 2015-16, 35 percent of all US youth were obese, up from 29 percent in 1999-2000. The prevalence of females aged 16 to 19 who were overweight or obese increased from 36 percent in 2013-14 to 48 percent in 2015-16. The prevalence of obesity among adults increased from 34 percent in 2007-8 to 40 percent in 2015-16. According to OECD statistics, obesity rates in the US are more than double those in continental Europe. While I know there are some who claim that "healthy obesity" is possible, I must stick with medical facts. Obesity is a huge contributor to ill health. Diabetes, coronary disease, high blood pressure, fatty liver, sleep apnea, many cancers and back and joint problems are all much higher in the obese. The CDC estimates that obesity-related diseases cost the nation $147 billion a year in health care-related expenses. Researchers from the University of Pennsylvania and the Boston University School of Public Health estimated that obesity in the US may be responsible for as many as 186,000 deaths a year, and that rising rates of obesity have shaved almost a year off our national life expectancy. When the whole planet is getting more obese, it is useless to blame the individual. The solution to obesity does not lie in the medical care system or in shaming individuals but in the social sphere. Healthier foods need to be easier to get and no more expensive than sodas and fries.

A telling story ran in *The Eagle Tribune*, a newspaper serving the Merrimac Valley in Massachusetts, in May 2018, headlined, "Group seeks better access to healthy foods in Lawrence." Lawrence is a small city, a former mill town that has a high percentage of its citizens living in poverty. The story noted that 82 percent of Lawrence residents live in a "food desert," lacking access to fresh produce and healthy foods. While there is a bodega (convenience store) on every corner, there are only three grocery stores to serve the 80,000 city-dwellers, and many residents lack transportation to get to them. The same story could be told about the inner cities around the country. Access to grocery stores, farmers markets and healthy food retailers has been linked to lower rate of obesity and diabetes, but for many poor people, this access is not available.

Recently published research showed that Canadians in "food insecure" households had over twice the rate of Type 2 diabetes as those in households with ready access to healthy food, and I assume the same holds true this side of the border.

The benefits of exercise are not restricted to marathon runners. It has been shown that as little as 30 minutes of brisk walking three times a week pays enormous dividends, but most of us still get in our cars to drive three blocks. We entertain ourselves by watching TV or playing video games rather than riding a bicycle or throwing a ball around.

One of the biggest reasons the death rate among teenagers in the US is so much higher than in the rest of the Western world is the very high rate of motor vehicle accidents, suicides and homicides. A study in the January 2018 issue of *Health Affairs* looked at death rates among children and teenagers in 16 developed OECD countries. US teenagers were 82 times more likely to die at the hands of a gunman than their peers in other countries.

In 2016, 38,658 people died of gunshots, of which 37 percent were homicides and 61 percent suicides, with two percent accidental. The means of suicide matter a very great deal. Most people who attempt suicide but survive get help and it is rare for them to repeat the attempt. When the means used is overdosing on pills or cutting their wrist, more than 90 percent survive a suicide attempt. When a gun is used for suicide, it results in death more than 90 percent of the time.

2018 has seen a school shooting somewhere in the United States on an average of once a week. While watching a cable news channel on a recent air trip, I saw a terrifying graphic. They listed the number of school shootings that had taken place from 2009 to date. The US tally was 288. In second and third place were Mexico and South Africa, with eight and six! After each tragedy, politicians mouth sanctimonious expressions of sorrow and then hop back into the pocket of the NRA. Nothing is done to prevent the next shooter from getting guns.

Despite some progress, more than 10,000 alcohol-related motor vehicle accident fatalities occur annually in the US. Every day, 29 people in the United States die in an alcohol-impaired driving crash.

Motor vehicle accidents are the leading cause of death for Americans aged 16 to 24 and the second-leading cause for children aged four to 15. More stringent state laws on alcohol have been shown to be associated with lower rates of alcohol-related driving fatalities. These laws target drinking-oriented policies, such as higher taxes on alcohol and limits on the density of alcohol sales outlets, and driving-specific policies, such as sobriety checkpoints and lower limits of blood alcohol at which DUI is invoked.

It will come as no shock to the reader when I say that we have a major problem with opioids. The CDC released a report in 2018 estimating that 72,000 people died of drug overdoses in 2017, two thirds of which were caused by opioids. Adults between the ages of 25 and 54, in the prime of life, had the highest rate of drug overdose deaths. The mortality rate (deaths per 100,000 people) from drug-use disorders in the US increased by an astonishing 618 percent between 1980 and 2014. Doctors who prescribe opioids and pharmaceutical manufacturers who push their use share in the blame for this gruesome statistic but cannot solve the problem without help from the legal system and society in general. Even as the opioid epidemic has become widely recognized and prescription use has fallen, illegal narcotics flood our country.

When will we reduce the access to guns that kill so many of our young people? When will we put teeth into stopping car accidents due to texting while behind the wheel? When will we severely punish those who drive while legally drunk?

Chapter 18

## One Possible Solution: Single Payer

As the US population ages, increases in health care spending will inexorably rise because of the greater demands of the elderly on the healthcare system. (People over 65 currently make up about 15 percent of the US population but account for about 31 percent of physician office visits.) It is imperative that we move as quickly as possible to control what we can control before health care expenditure bankrupts the country.

The Affordable Care Act, or "Obamacare," added some useful features that improved our current health insurance system. Probably the most important was to remove insurance companies' ability to disallow services related to pre-existing conditions. This exclusion from coverage was a major problem for the minority of adults who had developed a serious illness. It meant that if they lost their current insurance, they would no longer be able to get any health services related to that illness covered by their new insurance. It was a modern form of indentured service—leaving your company was playing Russian roulette with your health. Removing the lifetime cap on services was also important for the small number of patients with very expensive diseases, who through no fault of their own might find huge ongoing expenses no longer covered. The biggest problem with the ACA, in my opinion, was that it tried to improve or fine-tune our existing dysfunctional system. It did nothing to curb the rapacious practices I have outlined in previous chapters. It did nothing to try to bring down our outrageous health care costs. The American health insurance "system" remains a crazy quilt: superb health insurance for some, shaky high-premium, high-deductible insurance for others, and none for some 30 million of our fellow citizens. For many low-income workers, even with health insurance, health expenses can be a crushing burden. A careful analysis published in July 2018 looked at low-income families, defined as those with incomes less than twice the federal poverty level. During the 10-year study period ending December 2016, there were 8.2 million such families in which one or more members had atherosclerotic (coronary) heart disease. They faced mean annual out-of-pocket health costs of $2,227, including $722 for insurance premiums and $1,505 for medication, co-pays, etc. Of these families, 2.7 million paid more than 20 percent of their total income after subsistence (food) costs on health care and a million families faced catastrophic health care costs—meaning they had to spend more than 40 percent of their income after food on health care. And these were working people with health insurance!

Tinkering with our current system, as the ACA did, will not work. Even if we could get Congress to agree on a plan to expand coverage to all, which in the current climate seems impossible, the grossly overly-expensive costs associated with the current US non-system would not go down. The players in the system are acting in their own self-interest, with maximizing profit the chief motivator. For real improvement in affordable health care for America, we need much more dramatic steps.

The optimal solution, in my opinion and that of many others, is to move as quickly as possible to a single-payer system, AKA "Medicare for all." Let me note at this point that I am **not** a "socialist." My politics would be best described as those of a "Rockefeller Republican," fiscally conservative and socially liberal. I would love to believe that the "free market" could solve our problem, but I know that it will not and cannot. It is not socialist to believe that certain essential services are best provided by government rather than via the private sector. In most of the United States, police and fire protection are public services. The nation is protected by armed forces that are part of the federal government. Since our health and life are at stake, having an essential service such as basic health care should be guaranteed by our government.

The typical health insurance company takes about 12 to 13 percent of premiums for administrative costs and makes a profit as well. Medicare spends about 2 percent on administration! This comparison is a bit misleading because Medicare piggybacks off Social Security to handle enrollment and some other functions. Even so, at least 10 percent of total US health care spending could be immediately eliminated by switching to a single payer using the existing Medicare structure and cutting out the huge cost now going to private health insurers. If hospital and physician reimbursements were reduced to current Medicare levels, hospitals and doctors would be paid less, resulting in further savings. On average, Medicare pays about 78 percent of what commercial insurers pay doctors, so spending on physician fees would decrease. Since doctors would also see their billing and administrative costs dramatically cut, their net earnings would not be cut by nearly as much as their fees. The newly enlarged Medicare must be allowed to negotiate the price of pharmaceuticals. The price for medications could be cut by at least a third, cutting at least another five percent from our overall health care costs. These savings would generate more than enough to cover the cost of caring for the uninsured population and still leave major savings that could be spent on the many other needs facing the country.

This is not a new idea. Senator Bernie Sanders made it the key plank in his run for the presidential nomination. What is new is that doctors are increasingly comfortable with the idea. It was not that long ago that organized medicine was opposed to the original Medicare for seniors as "socialized medicine." A national survey of physicians conducted in 2008 by Merritt Hawkins found 58 percent of physicians opposed to single payer and 42 percent in favor. A newer survey conducted in 2017 found that 42 percent strongly support single payer and an additional 14 percent are somewhat supportive. Thirty-five percent strongly oppose the idea, 6 percent are somewhat against it, and 3 percent are undecided. Thus, in nine years, we have seen physician support for single payer grow from 42 percent to 56 percent.

There are many reasons for the shift. Part of it is generational, with younger physicians increasingly comfortable with the idea. Part of it is the growing frustration with the current "non-system" in which doctors seem to spend more time fighting insurance companies and filling out forms than they do caring for patients. Not surprisingly, primary care physicians are particularly in favor of single payer, as they are the most affected by the current mish-mash of rules and regulations.

While a growing majority of physicians are now in favor of single payer, most hospital executives remain opposed. As hospital reimbursements fall there are fewer insurance games to be played. The need for high priced administrators would fall, causing many to lose their jobs or see their salaries reduced. Health insurance and pharmaceutical industries are fervently against a plan that would lower their profits.

The biggest objection I hear to single payer is that our taxes would go up, as this, like current Medicare, would be a tax-funded program. While it is certainly true that federal taxes would go up, the overall amount spent would go down, and money currently spent on health insurance could be re-directed to our income. The overall balance for most Americans should be an increase in spendable income.

Another objection is that single payer systems in Great Britain and Canada result in long waits for needed services. We in the United States are used to getting every possible test, whether the test is needed or not, whenever we want it. As I discussed in the chapter on waste, much of this testing is not only a waste of money, it can be harmful. While it is true that it often takes longer to get elective surgery or non-urgent tests done in those countries, a large majority of the people in Canada and Great Britain are happy with their systems and have no interest in shifting to an American-style system. A poll conducted by the Toronto-based Nanos Research in April 2018 points to overwhelming support—86.2 percent—by Canadians for strengthening public health care rather than expanding for-profit services. The biggest problem in Canada and Great Britain is that overall health spending is kept too low for optimal service. They put 10 percent of their GDP into health care. We could opt to pay 12 percent and get more and prompter services. There is no reason why the United States could not adequately fund its health care system and still pay much less than it currently spends. I would also point out that expensive testing **is** rationed in the United States—but rationed by your insurance company rather than by a national health service.

Good friends of ours live in a major city in Canada. "Gloria" (not her real name) went to her primary care doctor for a persistent cough.

Her doctor sent her for a chest X-ray, which unfortunately was suspicious for lung cancer. Her care from that point involved a CT scan to better look at the lesion in the lung, followed by a PET scan, a biopsy, a consultation with a chest surgeon and cancer specialist, and then surgery. While each of these steps may have taken a few days longer than they would have in the United States, there was no serious delay, and her care was equal in every way to what she would have received in the United States. Her out-of-pocket cost for this care was only the optional charge she paid to have a single room while hospitalized. Gloria and her husband are certainly happy with Canada's single payer system.

Under a single payer system, people would be free, as they are in Canada, to buy supplemental insurance policies to cover non-covered services like cosmetic surgery or private rooms when hospitalized, and there would still be room for "concierge" doctors for those who wanted and could afford to pay for the extra service. Some co-pays could be included to encourage people to consider the cost and not feel that all the services they want are free. Those with the disposable income to afford more "upscale" service could buy it, just as they can buy luxury cars. For the large majority of Americans, these add-ons would not be needed or wanted, and the specter of losing your home or spending the money you had hoped to leave to your children because of a serious illness would be removed.

Gloria's case brought it home, but hers is not an isolated "best case scenario." A study presented at the annual meeting of the American Society of Clinical Oncology in June 2018 looked at the costs and outcomes of patients with advanced colorectal cancer treated on either side of the border—the province of British Columbia and the state of Washington. In many cases the patients lived within a few miles of each other. A total of $12,345 was spent per patient per month in Washington, while the corresponding figure in British Columbia was $6,195. The outcomes? The American patients survived an average of 21.4 months with active treatment while the Canadian patients survived slightly longer, at 22.1 months. In Canada you got results that were as good or better at half the cost.

There is no reason why a federally-mandated single-payer system need be monolithic like the British National Health Service. The Canadian system is structured around a federal mandate that necessary services such as hospital and doctors' services must be covered, but each province has wide latitude in how it administers the system within its borders. American states could be given the same latitude.

Who would win and who would lose under "Medicare for all?" The biggest winners would be the American public. While the Affordable Care Act has increased the numbers of people with health insurance, at least 29 million Americans are still uninsured. A report from the Commonwealth Fund in May 2018 found that the numbers of uninsured rose in 2016, reversing years of decline since the ACA was passed in 2010. With universal health care, there would be no more specter of bankruptcy from a serious illness. No more worrying if the doctors you want to see are covered under your plan. No more surprise charges. No more having to change doctors, hospitals or medications when the rules of your insurance changed.

Is single-payer health care perfect? No, but it is a huge improvement over our current non-system. *Business Insider* last summer posted a series of interviews with people who lived under a single-payer system, from Canada, Great Britain, Australia, Iceland and Finland. Their feelings echoed those of people around the world with whom I have spoken. Their complaints revolved around waits for non-emergency services and a degree of underfunding, but all were basically happy with their country's system, and each mentioned the freedom from worrying about the cost of medical care. There is no question that under our current system, Americans are used to getting what they want when they want it, while in Canada or other countries, there may be some delay in getting complex tests or elective surgery performed. However, it is very rare for an emergency test or procedure to be delayed. I have spoken to many Canadians, both doctors and patients, and have not heard of an urgently needed test being significantly delayed. There is always a trade-off between what services can be provided and what we as a country can afford. This is ultimately a political decision, whether we want to call it one or not. Under a single-payer system, these decisions could be made openly and rationally and the appropriate balance between health care and other societal needs would be a conscious decision and not just happen.

Primary care physicians would probably come out close to even financially. Their gross incomes would likely drop, but the accompanying drop in overhead would mean that net incomes would not decline as much, and most of the day-to-day hassles that make many doctors question why they went into medicine would be gone. The biggest losers would be the health insurance companies. There would doubtless be a role for them in processing Medicare claims, as there is now, but at a rate of no more than 2 percent plus expenses. Since they would be limited to simple claims processing, they would have to live within the much lower expense allowed by current Medicare. The pharmaceutical companies would see a drop in their enormous profits once a central insurer could negotiate prices. Hospitals also would suffer, as they generally fare better with commercial insurance rates than they do under Medicare. A 2014 survey by the American Hospital Association found that payments from commercial insurers covered 144 percent of hospital costs, while Medicare covered 88 percent. Their bottom line would not be as severely impacted, however, as the cost of billing for hospitals would also drop significantly. It also should be noted that what commercial insurers pay to hospitals for the same procedures varies widely. Prestigious hospitals can drive a hard bargain because the insurers want them "in network." They are typically paid almost twice the amount paid to small community hospitals based solely on prestige and marketing, rather than because they have better outcomes. Under Medicare, there is a differential higher payment schedule for teaching hospitals, since they employ residents and fellows, the practitioners of the future, and it is accepted that the cost of educating future doctors must be borne by those who will use their services in the future. However, the disparity in payments to major academic centers and community hospitals is not nearly as great as is the difference paid by commercial insurers, which is largely driven by the marketing clout of the academic centers rather than by any valid cost or quality differences.

Would switching to single-payer be easy? No—one does not turn an ocean liner on a dime, and one does not change a sector that makes up nearly 20 percent of the American economy overnight. There will need to be a phase-in, and compromises will be required along the way. Those who stand to lose money, including the health insurance industry, the pharmaceutical industry and the hospital industry, will fight tooth and nail to maintain their privileged status. We could start by allowing those younger than 65 to buy into existing Medicare, and encourage smaller employers and the self-employed to do this. Premiums would be based on an income-adjusted sliding scale. Once the politics are settled, the actual implementation would likely be easier than expected, because those doing the actual **work** of delivering health care would not change.

There would need to be a "grand bargain" between government and the private sector as employer-based and employer-paid insurance switched to a government-paid system. The huge amount of money freed up should not be used to boost the already-high salaries of CEOs or in share buy-backs. The lack of increase in employee earnings, despite record corporate profits in the current economic climate, tells us that companies will not be spontaneously generous. The enabling legislation that would shift health insurance costs away from employers would require either that this money be given to the employees in higher wages, who in turn would see part of it given up in higher taxes, **or** that corporate taxes would go up commensurate with the lower expenditures for health insurance so that in either instance this was not simply another windfall for corporate America.

The alternative of simply going on as we are doing is so frightening that a start must be made.

Chapter 19

## Other Steps to Take (With or Without Single Payer)

If single payer proves to be politically infeasible at the moment, there are intermediate steps that would help improve our costs and quality of care. Many of these could and should be implemented along with single-payer.

Legislation at either the federal or state level should require health insurers to offer a catastrophic health insurance policy. Patients would pay medical expenses up to 10 percent of their taxable incomes, and then the catastrophic policy would kick in to cover the rest. The Department of Health and Human Services should develop a model "basic" insurance plan that would cover the cost for physician and hospital services, including parity for mental health services, but which would not include the various mandated services that primarily increase costs. Patients would be required to pay their own bills until they hit the 10 percent cap, giving them a reason to question whether they really wanted the $2,000 MRI for their chronic back pain when the doctor said it was not needed. When we as patients "have some skin in the game" we are much more likely to be careful stewards of our health care spending. It would be crucial to include an annual cap on out-of-pocket expenses to protect lower income people. Co-pays and high deductibles are a much greater barrier to care for the poor than for the affluent. There would be no lifetime cap, so the victims of a serious illness would never worry about running out of insurance. This would allow health insurance to return to being insurance.

Federal subsidies should be used to lower the cost of medical school, so that repaying student loan debt is not a primary driver of graduates' choices. The reimbursement of primary care doctors should be raised and that of specialists lowered, so that graduates pick a field because of interest and not income. Make the incomes of most specialists and PCPs comparable, with any differential based on objective factors such as length of training or the added stress of longer work days and on call requirements. The system in which a doctor is paid much more for "doing something" to a patient rather than working with them to solve a problem simply leads to more "doing," even when the value is marginal.

Medicare and all other payers should introduce "site-neutral" payments. There is no reason to pay more for a test or procedure depending on where it is performed. If surgery can be performed safely in an outpatient "surgi-center," why pay more to have it done in a hospital?

The cost of medicines can and must be reduced through multiple actions. Most importantly, Congress should **immediately** amend the Medicare law to allow Medicare to negotiate with drug companies, as the VA now does. Unlike other government health care programs that fight for lower costs, Medicare is specifically barred by statute from so doing. The VA and the Department of Defense both pay an average of 24 percent less than other payers, using their ability to work with a limited formulary and large volume of purchases, and both Medicaid and a special program to help hospitals in low income areas (the 340B program) pay 23 percent less.

Make direct-to-consumer (DTC) advertising a non-tax-deductible cost for pharmaceutical companies. If the courts allow DTC ads as a form of "free speech," then force the ads to prominently include two key pieces of data now omitted: the actual size of the benefit (often not that great) and the retail cost of the medication. The FDA should prohibit patient coupon programs unless they are designed specifically to help low income patients and do not simply push patients into using more expensive medicines. Reduce the profit allowed on medications that have had their development cost largely subsidized by government research funding. The FDA should encourage the early entry of cost-saving generic drugs. The Justice Department should use anti-trust laws when a manufacturer is illegally trying to prevent the entry of competing generics.

CMS should immediately enlist the help of seniors in reporting fraud. Fines and penalties paid by offenders should be shared with the whistle blowers to encourage reporting of attempted fraud by doctors and patients.

Since much of the cost increase in health care is driven by scientific and technologic advancements (think MRI, angioplasty, robotic surgery), it is important to use neutral expert advice to assess how much these "advancements" improve patient outcomes while they are increasing costs. An example of the latter is robotic surgery for prostate surgery. This technology is heavily advertised by hospitals that offer it despite little evidence that it improves outcomes. Many new cancer drugs that come out are hugely expensive and extend life by just a matter of months, at the added personal cost of terrible side effects. My father had a wonderful saying: "Figures don't lie, but liars figure." I see this every day in claims about medical "advances." A new treatment is said to "significantly" extend life. This may be true in a statistical sense, but not in a way that is meaningful to patients and their families. An average time to death may be extended from nine to 10 months. With a large enough group studied, this may reach the commonly-used statistical cut-off of "less than 5 percent chance," that it was a fluke rather than being due to the treatment. Scientific papers are published and the pharmaceutical reps tout the "proven" benefits. What is lost in the hype is anything about quality of life or cost. Is the extra month of life really what patients would choose if they knew they would spend most of it vomiting? The Department of HEW should convene **neutral** panels to advise Medicare and other payers as to the suitability of new technologies for reimbursement.

Federal legislation should cap the administrative portion of what health insurers are allowed to spend at 8 percent of premiums. Insurers refer to what they pay in claims as their "loss ratio." This is the mind set—anything they pay to doctors and hospitals is a "loss," rather than their reason for existing. Instead, they should be allowed a reasonable amount to cover their expenses and not consider fancy suites for their executives a higher priority than paying the expenses of their insureds. Require all insurers to use a single credentialing and reimbursement mechanism. If every medical office and hospital used the same forms and procedures for billing, overhead costs would go down significantly. Require any disputes about whether a test or treatment is medically indicated to be decided by a neutral arbiter with no economic stake in the decision. Medical justification, and not the insurer's desire to keep costs down, should decide whether a test or procedure is needed.

CMS (Medicare) should convene panels of clinicians, health policy experts and patients to come up with a workable list of meaningful quality measures. These measures should include outcomes of importance to patients and reflect real health benefits. This list would be universally applied in any QA (quality assurance) programs by all who wish to do this form of measurement.

Common, expensive surgical procedures, such as heart surgery and joint replacement, should be paid on a "bundled" basis. The fee paid for the procedure should cover the entirety of care: pre-op, surgery and rehabilitation, as well as any re-admission for complications. This would give the surgeon and hospital incentives to use the best practices and not to drive up costs by doing unnecessary tests or save themselves money by getting the patient out of the hospital too quickly. Bundling has been shown to reduce costs, shorten lengths of stay and improve outcomes for cardiac surgery and for hip replacement. This method was going to be expanded from its trial basis until Tom Price took over as Secretary of HEW and canceled the planned mandatory program.

Before approving elective or invasive procedures, insurers should mandate the use of proven patient teaching aids that explain the pros and cons of the proposed procedure and allow adequate time for patients to get their questions answered, rather than simply handing them an unreadable consent form. Patients who receive adequate, unbiased advice are better able to give informed consent to proceed, or to decide against having the procedure.

Through public educational efforts, empower and encourage patients given a new diagnosis to ask basic questions without feeling that they are being "bad patients." They should ask the doctor the basis for the diagnosis and should also ask: "what else could it be?" If the doctor is not willing to answer these questions, patients should ask for another opinion, if not a new doctor.

Prioritize improving intercommunication between electronic medical record systems so that, with a patient's permission, the physician currently treating them can access all their medical information, no matter where care was received. Use available technology to enhance what doctors can do rather than simply replicating a paper chart on the computer. Numerous functions of the EMR can enhance care but have not been widely used because they do not fulfill various "mandates" and do not increase revenue.

At the state level, reform the malpractice system to a no-fault system in which patients harmed are reimbursed for expenses and lost wages and given a modest sum for pain and suffering. All cases should be heard in a tribunal headed by specially trained judges, eliminating the adversarial system with its exorbitant legal costs. When needed, medical experts should be hired by the tribunal and not be "hired guns" whose judgement is clouded by the source of their fees. If true malpractice was the cause of the harm, the hospitals and doctors involved should be referred for possible disciplinary action and retraining. A new model called CARe, for Communication, Apology and Resolution, has been tried in Massachusetts with success. After a patient injury, the physician who was involved or a hospital representative meets with the patient and family and explains what happened, expresses regret and lays out a plan for further care. If it appears that medical error was the cause of the injury, compensation is offered. A study of this method found that in most instances, standard of care **was** met, and it is helpful to the doctor(s) involved and the patient to know this. When the standard of care was not met, an apology and compensation is offered. This model led to early resolution of the problem in most cases and allowed the patient to continue care with the doctor should they wish, rather than becoming involved in legal action, which can last for up to seven years.

All levels of government must put money into practical efforts to reduce obesity and encourage more walking, bicycling and other healthy behaviors. We need to begin with our children and encourage regular exercise and healthy eating behaviors. Local governments can use incentives to encourage grocery chains to open in poorer neighborhoods so residents have access to healthy fruits and vegetables that are as easy to buy as the junk foods sold in convenience stores. The use of taxes and regulation to change behaviors needs to be investigated. Food manufacturers must reduce the amount of salt, fat, sugar and other unhealthy additives to their products.

One of the reasons so many European countries have better health status and lower health costs is that they have a better social support system and because activities such as riding a bicycle to work or to run errands are the norm. Although the US remains the world's richest country, it has the third-highest poverty rate among the OECD nations. Nearly one in every five American children live in a household described by the government as "food insecure," meaning they are without regular access to enough food for active healthy lives. Take some money from the health care profiteers and improve our school lunch programs!

Since the elderly use much more health care than younger people, we must improve our social support systems for our seniors. Americans are mobile, and we are not going to return to multigenerational families living together as the norm, so we need to offer more organized social services in the community. Preventing hospitalization by better support both improves the quality of life of elders and saves huge amounts of money.

Encourage patients with major life-threatening disease to have an in-depth conversation with their families and their doctors about what is important and whether they prefer to fight for every day or to prioritize comfort. These discussions should be held before a crisis ensues, and should be open and honest. If "every possible day longer" is the patient's wish, this should be honored, and so equally should their wish to place comfort and quality of life over a few extra weeks or months of discomfort. Having these discussions before a patient is in the emergency room or intensive care unit, with doctors poised to put a breathing tube down his windpipe, will spare patients and families much anguish.

A variety of methods have been proven to reduce deaths from alcohol-related motor vehicle accidents. These include higher taxes on alcohol, preventing the sale of alcohol to underaged persons and already intoxicated adults, enhanced law enforcement including sobriety checks, and ignition interlocks using a breath alcohol detector. The National Academy of Science published a lengthy report in 2018 that described these methods in detail. What is missing is not the means, but the will to use them.

Gun death rates vary dramatically among the states and correlate highly with state laws. Massachusetts has the lowest death rate from guns of any state, at 3.5 deaths per 100,000 people. If every state had the same rate of gun deaths as Massachusetts, 27,000 lives would be saved annually in the United States. In Massachusetts, all high-powered semiautomatic rifles and high-capacity magazines are banned for civilian use. All gun purchases, including private sales, require a background check. Local police decide who can own a gun, and laws allow police to remove guns from high-risk homes. Despite these restrictions, no one has their hunting rifles taken away. Hunting is alive and well in the Commonwealth, as can be testified by the many pick-ups parked off the highways during deer season and the enthusiastic recounting by some of my friends of their outings.

# Chapter 20

## The Future

We have a problem. Health care is enriching many people but bankrupting our country. Those who are least able to afford health care suffer the most and often have the poorest insurance coverage. Since we have the best Congress that money can buy, those who are profiting from the current system are willing to spend large sums of money to maintain the status quo. In Washington, DC, there are 20 registered lobbyists— many of whom represent the interests of the health care giants—for every member of Congress. Only if the American people stand up, speak loudly and make their wishes known at the ballot box will anything change.

There is nothing God-given or immutable about our current dysfunctional system. It is the product of years of lobbying by powerful interests and chance events. The powerful interests have been able to resist change because the American public has not considered health care to be a basic human right. Hopefully this is changing.

Members of Congress have wonderful health insurance at very low cost, so they do not feel the pain that most of us feel. Ironically, a tweet that went viral just before July 4, 2018—American Independence Day— captured the dilemma faced by everyday people. In Boston, a woman was severely injured when her leg was caught between a subway car and the platform. The cut went right down to bone. In agony, she begged bystanders not to call an ambulance, because she feared she could not afford it. Basic health care should be as much as a right as food and shelter, available to all who need it, not just to those who are lucky enough to be wealthy or have good health insurance.

While the inertia of keeping what we have combines with the monied interests to make major change difficult, change does occur in the United States when the people demand it. We have moved from Jim Crow laws to legal equality. We now recognize the rights of people who love each other to marry no matter what their race or gender. Harry Truman's proposal for Medicare went nowhere when he proposed it, only to be signed into law by Lyndon Johnson.

There are solutions. There are ways we can have better care at a lower price. Will we? Only we can decide.

Postscript

## Practical suggestions for immediate use

In the long run, for our own sake and for the sake of our children and grandchildren, major structural changes **must** be made in the delivery of health care in the United States. I hope I have convinced you of this and motivated you to begin working to see that these changes are made. In the immediate time frame, I have been asked to give you some ideas that you can put to practical use now.

Your costs for prescription drugs will never be **low,** but you can lower your costs in the following ways:

1. When a new medication is prescribed, ask if anything similar is available generically. You should print out and reference the Walmart Pharmacy list of drugs that they sell at $4 for a 30- or $10 for a 90-day supply and ask for medications on this list when they are appropriate for you. In many cases, this or other generic drug programs will give you your medication at a lower out-of-pocket cost than by using your insurance.

2. If your medication is a tablet, ask the doctor to prescribe a double-strength tablet that you can split. A 20 mg tablet is almost never priced at twice that of a 10 mg tablet.

3. Do not throw out prescription or over-the-counter medications because they have passed their expiration date. Pills and tablets are almost always effective for years after this date.

Online information can be good, mediocre or downright dangerous. When you want information about a disease or treatment, always start at the most trusted site—run by the National Institutes of Health: https://www.nih.gov/health-information. If you do not find what you need there, go to a site maintained by a large trusted hospital system such as the Mayo Clinic, Cleveland Clinic or Massachusetts General Hospital. If you do a Google search, remember that a high placement on the results page may mean that the site paid for placement and does not necessarily mean it is a high quality site.

Examine your hospital and doctor bills carefully. Look for duplicate charges and for charges for things that were not done.
There are many ways you can make a visit to the doctor more helpful:

1. Go prepared. Know what your goals are for the visit, which may or may not match the doctor's. For instance, you may be going to a visit that was scheduled to follow up on your hypertension or your diabetes, but you have developed a worrisome new symptom. Do **not** wait until the doctor is wrapping up the visit to bring up your new symptom. The "by the way" complaint makes life very hard on the doctor. Do they give this the attention it needs and put their schedule off for the rest of the session? Or do they try to brush it off, or ask you to schedule another visit? Do both the doctor and yourself a favor and begin the visit by voicing your main concern.

2. Bring notes and take notes. Have a check-list of important items such as any prescriptions that are running out and any problems that have occurred since your last visit. If new treatments are proposed or other recommendations are made, write these down. People forget most of what the doctor said almost as soon as they leave the office.

3. If you are seeing a new doctor, whether a specialist or primary care doctor, bring detailed information with you regarding your current medications and medication allergies, past surgeries, immunizations you have had, important family history and any recent tests you have undergone. Bring test results you have been given or have downloaded from a "patient portal." Do not assume doctors will be able to get these, as they often cannot.

4. If your doctor has scheduled a visit to follow-up after testing is done, call the office a day ahead to be sure the test results have reached the doctor. If they have not, the office staff will then have time to track down the results before your visit.

5. If you have sensory issues, particularly bad hearing or any memory issues, be sure to have a family member or friend accompany you, and perhaps act as your note-taker.

6. ASK QUESTIONS. There are no dumb questions, and you are being unfair to yourself if you get home and wish you had asked about something while you had the chance.

When you are given a new diagnosis, be prepared to ask the following questions, particularly if it is a serious condition or if you have been advised to start medication, have surgery or undergo invasive testing:

1. Why did you conclude that I have this condition, on what basis?

2. What else could it be and have you conclusively ruled out these other conditions?

3. How do you plan be sure? Do I need other tests or opinions?

4. If we are treating this new condition, when should I see improvement? When should I call or come in if I do not improve?

If it is a serious diagnosis or if major interventions are proposed, do not hesitate to ask for a second opinion. Good doctors should not be offended by this. Second opinions often change your care. Remember— it is the doctor's job to help you; it is not your job to make the doctor feel better by offering blind trust.

Have a current health care proxy and written advance directives. When you have serious medical issues or when you are simply old enough that such things may happen, it is important to think about what kind of care you would want if you are unable to speak for yourself. This is a very personal topic, and your wishes may well be different than someone else's. Is every moment your heart beats important to you, or is comfort more important than extra time? You should discuss this with your family and be sure they understand your choices. You want to have this discussion when you are in good condition, and not when a doctor is poised to insert a breathing tube in your throat. You also want your family to know they are carrying out your wishes and not put them in a position of making decisions that may or may not be those you would make. Putting all of this in writing is important, but so is talking, to make sure everyone is on the same page.

Look after yourself! Staying healthy is cheaper and better than dealing with preventable disease. Exercise regularly. Walk, swim, bicycle, garden – **move** your body at least 30 minutes most days of the week. It is good for your heart, your skeletal system, your brain and your mood. Eat your fruits and veggies. The occasional ice cream or pizza will not kill you; making fast food the staple of your diet may. If you drink alcohol, do so in moderation. That means up to 2 ounces of liquor (or 8 ounces of wine or two beers) for men and 1 ounce for women.

If you end up in the hospital, try to have a friend or family member with you as much of the day as possible. If permitted, have them get you up and walk frequently during the day. Sleep and adequate nutrition are an important part of the recovery process. If you find the food inedible, have foods you enjoy brought in. Ask your doctor to write an order specifying that you are not to be woken up at night for routine vital signs or pre-dawn blood draws.

References/Source Material

Introduction
www.healthsystemtracker.org/chart-collection/health-spending-u-s-compare-countries

How Cubans Live as Long as Americans at a Tenth of the Cost.
www.theatlantic.com/health/archive/2016/11/cuba-health/508859

http://www.commonwealthfund.org/publications/issue-briefs/2015/oct/us-health-care-from-a-global-perspective

https://www.statnews.com/2017/10/30/medical-debt-states

Child mortality in the US and 19 OECD comparator nations. Health Affairs 2018;37(1):140-149

Maternal mortality: https://www.usatoday.com/deadly-deliveries/interactive/how-hospitals-are-failing-new-moms-in-graphics/

Is the United States Maternal Mortality Rate Increasing? Obstet Gynecol 2016; 128(3): 447-455

Health care spending in the United States and other high-income countries. JAMA 2018; 319(10): 1024-1039

The anatomy of health care in the United States. JAMA 2013; 310(18): 1947-1963

http://www.marketwatch.com/story/this-is-the-harsh-reality-about-health-care-costs-in-retirement

https://www.reuters.com/article/us-usa-healthcare-worries/soaring-costs-loss-of-benefits-top-americans-healthcare-worries-ipsos-poll-idUSKBN1JB1FD

## Chapter 2
Health insurance coverage by occupation among adults 18-64. MMWR Weekly Report 2018; 67(21): 593-8

Health Insurance Coverage and Health- What the Recent Evidence Tells Us. New England Jl Medicine 2017; 377(6): 586593

Health Insurance and Mortality in US Adults. American Jl Public Health 2009; 99(12): 2289-95

A deadly wait for US health insurance: sitting on the couch with malaria. Am Jl Tropical Med and Hygiene 2018; 99(1): 24-26

Disparities in survival by insurance status in follicular lymphoma. Blood 2018. epub ahead of print. PMID 30042094

## Chapter 3
Re prices, in 2003
https://www.healthaffairs.org/doi/abs/10.1377/hlthaff.22.3.89

US vs Europe:
https://epianalysis.wordpress.com/2012/07/18/usversuseurope/

And in 2017:
https://jamanetwork.com/journals/jama/fullarticle/2661579

Factors associated with increases in US health care spending 1996-2013. JAMA 2017; 318(17): 1668-1678

Utilization rates of knee-arthroplasty in OECD countries. Osteoarthritis and Cartilage. 2015; 23: 1664-1673

## Chapter 4
www.cms.gov/research-statistics-data-and-systems

## Chapter 5

https://www.nytimes.com/2014/05/18/sunday-review/doctors-salaries-are-not-the-big-cost.html

https://www.npr.org/sections/health-shots/2018/05/25/613685732/why-your-health-insurer-doesnt-care-about-your-big-bills

Prior authorization reform for better patient care. JACC 2018; 71(17): 1937-1939

A health care paradox: measuring and reporting quality has become a barrier to improving it. https://www.statnews.com/2017/12/13/health-care-quality/

Disentangling health care billing for patients' physical and financial health. JAMA 2018; 319(7): 661-663

Measuring the burden of health care costs on US families. JAMA 2017; 318(19): 1863-1864

Potentially avoidable emergency department use: when policy expects patients to be physicians. Annals of Emergency Medicine 2018. epub ahead of print.

Absolute Insurer Denial of Direct-acting Antiviral Therapy for Hepatitis C: A National Specialty Pharmacy Cohort Study. https://academic.oup.com/ofid/article-lookup/doi/10.1093/ofid/ofy076

## Chapter 6

https://www.nytimes.com/2017/10/25/upshot/the-unhealthy-politics-of-pork-how-it-increases-your-medical -costs
https://catalyst.phrma.org/how-much-are-hospitals-marking-up-the-price-of-medicine-the-answer-may -surprise-you

Politics, hospital behavior and health care spending. The National Bureau of Economic Research. NBER working paper 23748. Issued August 2017

Hospitals employing physicians:
http://www.physiciansadvocacyinstitute.org/PAI-Research/Physician-Employment-Impact-on-Medicare-Spending

Billing errors: https://www.newsmax.com/health/health-news/medical-bill-error-mistake/2017/08/04/id/805882

Chapter 7
Health Affairs Volume 36, No. 1

https://www.vox.com/2018/5/23/17353284/emergency-room-doctor-out-of-network

Variation in physician charges by specialty: JAMA 2018; 317(3): 35-6

Chapter 8
Mortality and Treatment Patterns Among Patients Hospitalized with Acute Cardiovascular Conditions During Dates of National Cardiology Meetings. JAMA Internal Medicine 2015; 175(2): 237-244

https://www.statnews.com/2017/09/05/rising-debt-medical-school

Where have all the generalists gone? They became specialists, then subspecialists. American Jl Med 2017; 130(7): 766-768

https://www.nytimes.com/2017/06/03/opinion/sunday/the-specialists-stranglehold-on-medicine.html

The importance of continuity of care:
https://bmjopen.bmj.com/content/bmjopen/8/6/e021161.full.pdf

Chapter 9
https://www.gallaghermalpractice.com/state-resources/massachusetts-medical-malpractice

Re hiding errors: Am J Clin Pathol. 2018; 149: 458-460

Medical errors, malpractice and defensive medicine: an ill-fated triad. Berlin L. Diagnosis 2017; 4(3): 133-139

Caps lead to less invasive testing: Farmer SA et al JAMA Cardiology. epub 6/6/2018

Less defensive medicine when no liability concerns: Frakes MD, Gruber J. NBER Working Paper 24846 July 2018

**Chapter 10**
www.drugcostfacts.org/us-healthcare-spending

re neratinib: JAMA 2018; 319(21): 2167-8

re deflazacort: JAMA Neurology 2018; 75(2): 143-144

delayed generic adoption: JAMA Internal Medicine 2018;178(5):721-2

Why drugs cost more in the US than Mexico: American Jl Medicine 2015; 128(12): 1265-7

Pharma lobbying: www.statnews.com/2017/12/19/pharma-lobbying-spending/

Making Medicines Affordable: A National Imperative. National Academies Press. 2017

Research and development spending to bring a single cancer drug to market and revenues after approval. JAMA Internal Medicine 2017; 177(11): 1569-75

A much-needed corrective on drug development costs. JAMA internal Medicine 2017; 177(11): 1575-6

Selling Patents to Indian Tribes to Delay the Market Entry of Generic Drugs. JAMA Internal Medicine. Published online January 2, 2018

https://www.cnn.com/2018/06/29/health/acthar-mallinckrodt-medicare-claims-doctor-payments/index.html

Conflicts of interest in FDA panels:
http://www.sciencemag.org/news/2018/07/hidden-conflicts-pharma-payments-fda-advisers-after-drug-approvals-spark-ethical

Limited evidence supporting FDA fast-tracking: JAMA 2018; 320(3): 301-303

NIH Funding supports drug development: www.pnas.org/cgi/doi/10.1073/pnas.1715368115

Chapter 11
Schulman KA, Richman BD: The evolving pharmaceutical benefits market. JAMA 2018; 319(22): 2269-2270

Which firms profit most from America's health-care system. The Economist. May 15, 2018

http://www.dispatch.com/news/20180519/powerful-secretive-middlemen-affect-drug-prices

Chapter 12
The High Cost of Unnecessary Care. JAMA 2017; 318(18): 1748-9

Overtreatment in the United States. PLoS One 2017; 12(9): e018970

Comparison of Lab testing in teaching vs. nonteaching hospitals. JAMA Internal Medicine 2018; 178(1):1-6

2017 Update on medical overuse. JAMA Internal Medicine 2018; 178(1): 110-115

Localized prostate cancer: treatment options. American Family Physician 2018; 97(12):798-805

Impact of clinical practice guidelines on use of intra-articular hyaluronic acid and corticosteroid injections for knee osteoarthritis. J Bone Joint Surg America 2018; 100: 827-834

Futility of anticonvulsants in treating pain: CMAJ 2018 July 3;190:E786-93. doi: 10.1503/cmaj.171333

Chapter 13
https://www.bostonglobe.com/metro/2018/05/24/doctor-lawsuit-says-steward-health-care-pressured-doctors-to-restrict-referrals-outside-chain

http://khn.org/news/fraud-and-billing-mistakes-cost-medicare-and-taxpayers-tens-of-billions-last-year

https://www.snopes.com/fact-check/did-cdc-flu-shot-causing-outbreak/

Chapter 14
Improving end of life discussions: Curtis JR et al. JAMA Internal Medicine 2018. May 26. epub ahead of print.

Factors contributing to geographic variation in end-of-life expenditures for cancer patients. NL Keating et al. Health Affairs 2018. Volume 37.

Effect of early palliative care on chemotherapy use and end-of-life care in patients with metastatic non-small-cell lung cancer. J Clin Oncol 2011; 30: 394-400

Predictors of hospice enrollment for patients with advanced heart failure and effects on health care use. J Am Coll Cardiol HF 2018 epub ahead of print

Chapter 15
The "bible" on diagnostic error: Balogh E, Miller BT, Ball JR, eds.: Improving Diagnosis in Health Care. National Academies Press, 2015

Physicians' Diagnostic Accuracy, Confidence, and Resource Requests. JAMA Internal Medicine 2013; 173(21): 1952-9

Value of second opinions:
https://www.mayoclinicproceedings.org/article/S0025-6196(14)00245-6/pdf

Chapter 16
EMR frustration: JAMA Internal Medicine 2018; 178(6): 741-2

www.dotmed.com/legal/print/story.html?nid=43147

Alert fatigue: www.bostonglobe.com/metro/2018/06/06/brockton-hospital-staff-overlooked-warning

Relationship Between Clerical Burden and Characteristics of the Electronic Environment with Physician Burnout and Professional Satisfaction. Mayo Clinic Proc 2016; 91(7): 836-848

Re physician "burn-out:" https://www.medscape.com/slideshow/2018-lifestyle-burnout-depression-6009235

Relation between physician burnout and medical errors: https://www.mayoclinicproceedings.org/article/S0025-6196(18)30372-0/fulltext

Nurses' workarounds in acute healthcare settings: a scoping review. BMC health Services Research 2013; 13:175-191

Analysis of errors in dictated clinical documents assisted by voice recognition software. JAMA Network Open 2018; 1(3):e180530

Clinical documentation in the 21st century. Ann Intern Med 2015; 162:301-303

Resolving the productivity paradox of health information technology. JAMA 2018; 320(1):25-26

Weed LL. Medical records that guide and teach. N Engl J Med 1968; 278:593-600

## Chapter 17

Re American diet: JACC Heart Failure 2017:5(9):686-7

Obesity: http://time.com/5100737/obesity-lowering-life-expectancy-united-states

Prevalence of obesity among adults. MMWR Weekly reports 2017; 66(50):1369-73

http://www.eagletribune.com/news/merrimac_valley/group-seeks-better-access-to-healthy-foods-in-lawrence

Youth Risk Behavior Surveillance – United States 2017 MMWR Weekly Reports 2018; 67(8):1-114

Trends and patterns of geographic variation in mortality from substance use disorders and intentional injuries among US counties, 1980-2014. JAMA2018; 319(10):1013-1023

Relationship of alcohol consumption to all-cause, cardiovascular and cancer-related mortality in US adults. JACC 2017; 70(8):913-922

Death by gun violence – a public health crisis. JAMA internal Medicine 2017; 177(12):1724-5

Fighting unarmed against firearms. JAMA Network Open Access 2018; 1(3):e180845

Influence of lifestyle on incident cardiovascular disease and mortality in patients with diabetes mellitus. JACC 2018; 71(25):2867-2876

Follow up after unsuccessful suicide attempts: Comparison of the safety planning intervention with follow-up vs usual care of suicidal patients treated in the emergency department. JAMA Psychiatry 2018.1776. Published online July 11, 2018

## Chapter 18

Which road to universal coverage? New England Jl Med 2017; 377(23):22072209

A single-payer system: Best for doctors and patients alike? http://www.medscape.com/viewarticle/855269

The virtues and vices of single-payer health care. New England Jl Med 2016; 374(15):1401-1403

http://nymag.com/daily/intelligencer/2016/05/medicare-for-all-isnt-as-easy-as-it-sounds.html

Association of out-of-pocket annual health expenditures with financial hardship in low-income adults with atherosclerotic cardiovascular disease in the United States. JAMA Cardiology 2018; 1813. Published online July3, 2018

5 people from around the world share what it's like to have single-payer healthcare. http://www.businessinsider.com/what-single-payer-healthcare-is-like-2017-8

https://catalyst.nejm.org/clinicians-support-single-payer-win-lose/

Lack of salary gains despite increased corporate profits:
https://www.nytimes.com/2018/07/13/business/economy/wages-workers-profits.html?emc=edit_th_180714&nl=todaysheadlines&nlid=602372910714

## Chapter 19
www.commonwealthfund.org/publications/blog/2016/may/drug-price-control-how-some-government-programs-do-it

Association of state alcohol policies with alcohol-related motor vehicle crash fatalities among US adults. JAMA internal Medicine 2018. Published online May 29, 2018

Getting to Zero Alcohol-impaired Driving Fatalities. The National Academies Press. 2018

## Chapter 20
Congressional health coverage:
https://www.cnbc.com/2017/07/25/heres-how-much-members-of-congress-pay-for-their-health-insurance.html

This tweet captures the state of health care in America today. Editorial. New York Times, July 3, 2018

# Acknowledgements

Many people helped me complete this book. Special thanks to colleagues Mitch Feldman, MD, and Greg Estey of the MGH Lab of Computer Science; Ruth Ryan, Secretary of the Society to Improve Diagnosis in Medicine (SIDM); and Mark Graber, MD, President of SIDM, who reviewed early drafts and made helpful suggestions. David Himmelstein, MD, pointed out a few discrepancies in my numbers, which I corrected, and made other useful suggestions.

Friends Tom and Barbara Farquhar, Jim and Pat Poitras and my son Scott carefully read the manuscript and offered a "patient's-eye" perspective, pointing out areas where I needed to be clearer or more descriptive for the non-medical reader. I talked out many of the issues with my son Jed. Thanks to my editor, Theresa Driscoll, for toning down some of my too-florid prose, and to Henry Quinlan, head of Omni Press, who encouraged me to complete the book.

Special thanks to my beloved wife and life partner, Pamela, who suffered through numerous revisions and caught many typos and other errors.

Any failings are my own.

## About the Author

Edward Hoffer, MD, graduated from the Massachusetts Institute of Technology with a degree in Economics, Politics and Science. He graduated Magna cum Laude from Harvard Medical School in 1969 and completed four years of postgraduate training at the Massachusetts General Hospital. He worked in one of the first Health Maintenance Organizations in the east, the Harvard Community Health Plan, for two years and then served as the Director of Ambulatory Services at Memorial Hospital in Worcester, MA. From 1978 through 2017 he was in solo or small group practice of Cardiology and General Internal Medicine.

Dr. Hoffer has held multiple administrative and leadership roles, including Medical Director of the Office of Emergency Medical Services of the Massachusetts Department of Public Health, President of the Middlesex West Medical Society, Vice President of the Medical Staff at Framingham Union Hospital, Medical Director of Hospice at Home (Wayland, MA) and President of Framingham Cardiology Diagnostics. He has also held, through the present, a part-time position at the Massachusetts General Hospital's Laboratory of Computer Science, working in the broad field of medical informatics, which uses computer technology to improve medical care. He is Treasurer and a Board member of the Society to Improve Diagnosis in Medicine (SIDM) and is Associate Professor of Medicine, part-time, at Harvard.

Dr. Hoffer's career has spanned a time of enormous change in the science and practice of medicine. While the science has dramatically improved, the process of delivering that science to patients has not. Focus has moved away from caring for the sick and into delivering profits to corporations. Burn-out has become epidemic among doctors who feel less and less able to do what prompted them to go to medical school: to care for the sick.

Made in the USA
Middletown, DE
17 September 2018